jailhouse

A TRIBUTE TO MY PATIENTS

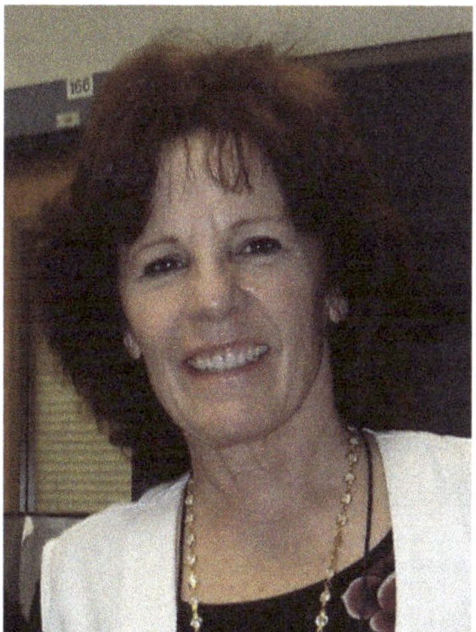

Nancy Smith, RN

Jailhouse is a work of nonfiction.

Names and identifying details have been changed.

Library of Congress Cataloging-in-Publication Data

Smith, Nancy

Jailhouse / by Nancy Smith

Includes index.

ISBN: 979-8-9970677-0-0

Printed in the United States of America

Praise for Jailhouse

Good Read

The author did an amazing job of detailing a nurse's life "on the inside". I would recommend this book to every nurse and nursing student. The diversity of what a jail nurse does is beyond imagination! Kudos to Nancy Smith.

Amazing!

If you are looking for a good read, this is it! So good. I hope there is more coming, because I want to know all the stories.

Well Written

I recommend this book to everyone to read. These stories provide insight into what nurses in correctional settings have to go through.

Insightful

Anyone who does your job deserves a medal of honor. I know I wouldn't do it. They are lucky to have someone compassionate to help them in their time of need.

Great Book

These books should be required reading for all medical practitioners and administrators working in jails or prisons. They certainly belong on the shelf of every nurse, physician, ancillary healthcare professional, and corrections administrator.

Inspiring

An inspiring book for our troubling times. It has never been more important to care for one another. Correctional nurses deal with a population of disadvantaged and vulnerable patients at a difficult time in their lives. Over two million incarcerated patients need you.

Compassion

Let's be thankful for wonderful nurses and caregivers who inspire us to recognize how we treat people, how we speak to them, and what we do that heals.

WOW

I really enjoyed this book. For those who love reading. It was honest. I liked the inclusion of quotes scattered throughout.

Well written and interesting.

Truly fascinating stories about real situations. Heartbreaking, mesmerizing, and shocking. Absolutely recommend this read.

Contents

Jailhouse

> ***When I grow up, I want to help inmates be as healthy as they can be !***
>
> — *said no kid, ever*

Correctional nursing was never part of my plan, but stepping into Oakwood changed me. Beneath the noise, steel, and guarded faces, I found unexpected humanity—complex, vulnerable, and often misunderstood. Behind bars, compassionate care thrives in ways the public never sees. I began writing down what I saw because the events I witnessed could no longer stay only in my heart.

Let me introduce myself. My name is Nancy Smith. I never imagined my nursing journey would lead me, decades into my career—which spanned the polished corridors of modern hospitals, acute care, home care, and the hushed farewells of hospice—to a place defined by razor wire, steel doors, strict rules, and locked gates: jail, a correctional facility.

Correctional nursing is a necessary specialty. It is not simply about administering medications or taking vitals. It's about providing quality healthcare to one of the most marginalized populations in society: incarcerated individuals. When an inmate enters jail or prison, access to health care does not (and should not) go away. In fact, for many, it's the first time they've seen a doctor in years.

Countless inmates enter the system with serious, untreated conditions—chronic illnesses, mental health issues, addiction, and a backlog of neglect from years without adequate medical attention. Many arrive with untreated diabetes, high blood pressure, festering wounds, broken teeth, mental illness, addiction—ghosts of a life without access to medical care, much less general stability. Behind bars, sickness doesn't pause. Illness doesn't care if you're wearing orange. Inmates wrestle with everything from chronic disease to the raw anguish of withdrawal, from deep psychological wounds to simple infections that fester in the silence. For some, the attention of a nurse is the first human kindness they've received in a long time. Many inmates have grown accustomed to having had little to no access to consistent healthcare in the outside world. For them, even basic medical care can feel like a lifeline—and they value it.

Before I entered the gates of Oakwood Correctional Facility, I had built a solid foundation in nursing: 25 years of experience in acute care, home health, and hospice. I'd sat beside lonely veterans in VA hospitals, watched families say goodbye to loved ones in hospice, and managed crises over the phone in the dead of night.

One day, while in a home care patient's poorly maintained home, I was sitting on newspaper on a filthy couch, helping him manage his medication regimen. I tried to remain calm when, out of the corner of my eye, I spied a foot-long rat running along the wall.

Years later, with the protection of sheriff deputies, I found myself beside a jail inmate whose face had just been slashed in an act of retaliation—blood pooling at his feet. That moment, among countless others, taught me this work is unlike anything else in mainstream nursing. Nothing quite prepared me for the intense, unpredictable, and often profoundly human experiences I would have in my time as a correctional nurse.

After a few years at Oakwood, it struck me: the public knows little about what really happens inside jails. Correctional healthcare is often invisible. What little the public sees is filtered through sensationalized television and headlines. Gangs. Violence. Lockdowns. These only tell part of the story. What's missing are the moments of compassion, healing, and quiet resilience. The quiet moments. The unexpected laughter. The inmate who offers you a drawing. The deputy who ensures your safety. The mental health counselor who gently coaxes someone through a panic attack. Inside Oakwood, something in me shifted. The noise, the echoing steel, the faces trying to mask fear with bravado —it all pressed in on me. Yet beneath that hardness, I felt a pulse of humanity I couldn't ignore. I discovered a level of humanity, complexity, and vulnerability that contrasted with public misconceptions, revealing the reality of a compassionate, complex healthcare system existing behind bars. I found people aching to be seen, stories begging to be understood, and a world far more complex than the public realizes. I began writing these memories because my heart could no longer hold them.

These are the stories I want to tell. So, I started writing them down—short stories, true stories. Each one is a snapshot of life behind the walls. Some are intense. Some are tender. All are real.

These stories spotlight the deeply human interactions among inmates, medical doctors, nurses, mental health professionals, deputies, chaplains, and correctional administrators. Sometimes they show the drama of crisis, yes—but more often, they show unlikely moments of connection. A deputy wipes blood off a man's face. Mental health staff hold steady during a psychotic break. A chaplain and a medic stand side by side in grief.

These tales often center on a specific medical issue. Sometimes, they reflect a collaboration between medical and mental health teams. Other times, they show how custody staff play a surprisingly compassionate role in inmate care.

This book isn't a traditional memoir. There's no central protagonist. Just a series of windows, each one offering a glimpse into the complex, chaotic, and surprisingly compassionate world of correctional care.

You'll read about trauma and survival, withdrawal and recovery, brutality and unexpected beauty. Some of it will be hard to take. I've witnessed high-adrenaline scenarios—cell extractions, crisis interventions—but I didn't want this book to just be a compilation of dramatic scenes. Yes, terrible things can happen in jail—but so do acts of grace, kindness, and healing.

My goal is to highlight the humanity that exists within those walls. Good people working in the corrections setting make a difference every day. I hope these stories add perspective to the way the general public thinks of life behind bars.

Some of the stories ahead may contain unpleasant, graphic content, but they reflect the reality of my experiences.

Nancy Smith – My Life in Nursing

I always knew I was meant for healing. Nursing shaped me through every loss and every life saved. When a coworker jokingly suggested working at the jail, I laughed—but I still applied for a position. That moment led to 16 years at Oakwood, where unpredictability and transformation became daily life. Oakwood didn't just change me—it rewired me.

When I was just 8 years old, my neighbor was a pathologist at our local county hospital. One weekend day, he asked his daughter and me if we wanted to go for a ride. "Want to come with me while I check some tissue samples?"

Of course, we said yes. A ride in his old Volvo, a walk through a maze of courtyards, and suddenly I was standing outside the lab, completely enchanted. The scent of aged trees mixed with antiseptic hung in the air. The building looked ancient and important. I didn't know what a hospital *really* was yet, but I knew one thing: I wanted to work here when I grew up!

Fast forward nearly a dozen years: two years after high school, I landed my first job as a nurse's aide on the surgical ward of that very hospital, which had become a full-fledged Medical Center. And wouldn't you know it, that same smell was still there—the comforting mix of bleach, linoleum, and something unexplainable.

The surgical floor also housed the Jail Ward. It was just four rooms, each with two hospital beds, and a deputy would sit in the hallway at all times when an inmate was present. "They never take the shackles off," one of the senior nurses told me during orientation. Sure enough, every inmate was cuffed to their bed. The deputy came with us every time we stepped inside.

I remember one inmate with hollow eyes and a raspy breath. It was a nighttime shift. "Got shanked in the yard," the deputy muttered. "Suffered a collapsed lung." It was my first encounter with the gritty side of healthcare. I didn't realize then that years later, I would close out my nursing career back in corrections.

My nursing path took me far and wide. My first role as an RN was still at that Medical Center—on a mixed floor that handled everything: ortho, ENT, GU, and overflow surgeries. It was trial by fire. I loved that place so much, I refer to it as "my beloved Medical Center."

Eventually, I moved to Los Angeles, and the first thing I did was look up the local county hospital. "If I'm going to work anywhere," I thought, "it'll be there." I got the job—and the experience—but after a year, I needed a change. So I applied at the VA hospital next.

"Always remember," the orientation nurse said firmly, "you're here to care for our veterans."

I carried that phrase with me. Caring for them was an honor. It was also exhausting; monthly rotating shifts meant only one precious month of days before swinging back to nights or evenings. Still, the work was meaningful.

Next, I found myself in home care. Driving the wild streets of L.A., I stepped into homes full of stories and struggle. Patients who were recovering from surgery or managing chronic conditions. It felt intimate. Personal. Real. "I'm glad it's you," a woman with congestive heart failure once told me, her hand resting lightly on mine. "You don't treat me like a number." Those moments are why I stayed.

Later, I followed a brilliant mentor to a hospital closer to my home in the San Fernando Valley. My commute dropped to fifteen minutes. "I actually giggle on my way to work," I told her one morning. And it was true.

Eventually, she helped me land one of the first remote positions—doing quality control on home care charts from my living room. In the *1980s*! I couldn't believe I was getting paid to sit at my kitchen table with a cup of coffee and a stack of records.

Moving back to the San Francisco Bay Area, I shifted into hospice care. It was emotionally heavy work, but some of the most meaningful I'd ever done.

I came to the Oakwood correctional nursing job as kind of a joke. I was working in hospice/homecare when a hospice coworker suggested we apply for part-time jobs at the jail. She seemed sure that it would be pretty easy work.

"Let's get jobs at the jail," my coworker said one day over lunch, grinning.

"You're kidding," I said.

"Nope. Easy work, part-time. Think about it."

And I did. I applied half out of curiosity—got the job, and stayed for sixteen years. At first, it was all new: diabetic calls, pill calls, detox assessments. But that wasn't all.

"Medical to D-Pod, man down!" the radio would crackle. And then it began—again.

It could be anything: a seizure, chest pain, full-blown heart attack, labor, or a fight gone wrong. Sometimes it was real. Sometimes...not so much.

"I think I'm dying," one inmate groaned, clutching his side.

"Okay," I said calmly, taking his vitals. "Tell me where it hurts."

He peeked one eye open. "Do I still get a treat if I go to the ER?"

Yeah. Not dying.

I spent the first few years learning my job. There were the routine parts of the job: the diabetic calls, pill calls, and assessments; the blood pressure checks, wound care, and assessments of patients detoxing from ETOH and drugs. But in between the routine were lots of interruptions in the form of "man-downs"—everything from full-blown myocardial infarctions to active labor, raging hypertension, and altercations, to the "pretend" events I mentioned.

The deputies would call for Medical to assess an inmate who was exhibiting symptoms of a medical problem. When the nurse arrived, an assessment would be carried out: a history of symptoms, vital signs, and other medical information. Experiencing these unexpected events during my shift started to affect me in ways I didn't realize right away.

The job came with a different kind of pressure. Over time, I noticed I started prepping for my shift like I was going into battle. My heart rate would pick up. My senses sharpened.

"I don't get that feeling anymore," I said to my husband recently while we watched the TV show *Emergency*. "But I remember it." The adrenaline. The readiness. The alertness that becomes second nature.

Working in a jail changes you. You learn to clock exits, scan faces, and watch for weapons improvised from everyday items like paper clips or socks. Safety is not a given—it's something you *ensure*. And still, every day, I loved the work.

The inmate population has changed since I started. What was once a population of mostly substance users has shifted—now about 50% of inmates have diagnosed mental illnesses. The passage of AB109 added more former prison inmates to local jails. Then came oversight from the Prison Law Office. Better care. Better living conditions. And—believe it or not—biweekly movie nights, complete with popcorn and soda.

I retired recently. Sixteen years in corrections, ending a lifetime in nursing. Which had all started with a walk outside a lab, in the shadow of old brick buildings, under whispering trees.

> ***The purpose of life is not to be happy.***
> ***It is to be useful, to be honorable,***
> ***to be compassionate, to have it***
> ***make some difference that you***
> ***have lived and lived well.***
>
> *- Ralph Waldo Emerson*

Oakwood Correctional Facility

Oakwood evolved from a 19th-century almshouse into a complex, often tense modern jail. More than a building, it felt alive—tense and unpredictable. Working among the mentally ill and the forgotten forced me to confront myself and understand how deeply safety and healthcare intertwine. I grew stronger, gentler, and braver, learning its rhythms and how quickly silence could turn to violence.

In the 1870s, the acreage that would later become Oakwood was owned by a farmer who raised thoroughbred horses and built a Victorian mansion on the estate. The County bought the property for $24,000 in 1884 and began using it as an almshouse: a shelter for the poor, forgotten, and impoverished, prompting residents to dub the mansion the "palace for the poor." The site became a compassionate haven for the homeless to live and work on the farm, planting, growing, and harvesting crops. They then sold those crops, providing the homeless with meaningful employment and some funds for food and shelter.

In the 1950s, the County began using the almshouse to house low-risk prisoners, establishing what would become the Oakwood Correctional Complex. When area residents wanted to incorporate as a city, they faced a dilemma because the law required a minimum population of 500, but the town had only 400 residents. Oakwood had an equal-sized population. Thinking outside the box, the County allowed the Oakwood inhabitants to be counted, which enabled city incorporation in 1954.

An aerial view of the property illustrating the layout of buildings, along with abbreviations, acronyms, and nomenclature, is included in the next chapter: Compendium. *This is a handy reference of terms used throughout this book.*

Oakwood Correctional Facility has since expanded into a primary county detention center that houses about 2,100 male and 500 female inmates on any given day. Men and women are housed in separate buildings, and separate wings with capabilities for medium- and minimum-security prisoners. Minimum security inmates are housed dormitory-style, with bunk beds. Oakwood employs approximately 300 County Department of Corrections (Office of the Sheriff) officers and 25 administrative support staff.

Inmate housing is divided according to an inmate's security level. The Classification staff interviews each inmate and selects housing either based on one's charges or behavior. Murder and attempted murder mean maximum security. There is maximum security housing on-site for women, but max security men are not housed at Oakwood. Officers have told me that inmates charged with robbery, fraud, and drug charges are assigned to Lockdown. Meanwhile, some inmates with lesser charges can have a high security classification because of assaultive behavior involving the staff.

Protective custody is another class. These are inmates with charges of child molestation or elder abuse, at-risk inmates (elderly, debilitated), and inmates who believe someone wants to hurt them in jail. It is my understanding that inmates can request protective custody because of their charges, their age, their sexual orientation, or their gang affiliation. When I started working at Oakwood, one building was used to house Protective Custody inmates. Fifteen years later, there are several more. Certain groups of gang members are also housed in protective custody to keep them away from rival gang members. And some inmates must be housed alone because they do not get along with anyone!

The largest population of inmates is housed in an area referred to as "minimum," for those with less serious charges waiting to be sentenced. The minimum area also contains men rehoused from prison under AB109. This means a very sophisticated inmate previously in prison might be housed with a kid who was just moved from Juvenile Hall on his 18th birthday!

Oakwood has changed quite a bit over the last five years. Violence between the inmates and deputies has increased. When AB 109 was passed in 2011 to help solve California's prison overcrowding problem, inmates ended up being supervised by the local probation and Sheriff where they were originally arrested. These were non-violent, non-serious, and non-sex offenders who would serve their time in local or county jail rather than the state prisons. According to deputies, very sophisticated criminals from prison are now mixed in with youngsters arrested for the first time. The resulting level of violence gives Medical and Mental Health staff nightmares.

Once the California Department of Corrections (DOC) inmates were returned from prison to Oakwood to relieve the prison overcrowding problem, the deputies had to step up their game. There had ALWAYS been drugs in jail, but now the deputies warned us to be much more careful when we were around them. In recent years, deputies have started wearing body cameras in inmate housing areas to improve safety and security.

Oakwood jail houses women in custody, approximately 500, at all security classifications. One building houses the minimum and medium security ladies. The other women's building houses the Special Management ladies (ladies with Mental Health diagnoses) in one dorm, while another dorm there houses ladies who must be in single & double cells because of their charges and/or their inability to get along with anyone else, as well as the ladies who have been charged with serious crimes. Many of these ladies are charged with crimes like murder, but they have demonstrated an ability to get along with others. These ladies stay with us for years as their cases wind through the courts. The initial drama they may have exhibited is replaced with a pretty laid-back attitude. The last dorm in this building has only individual cells. These ladies here are housed for a variety of reasons not revealed to the medical staff.

A correctional facility is an institution where individuals convicted of crimes are detained. It serves as a place for incarceration, rehabilitation, and punishment of offenders. County facilities are jails where, in general, an offender is sentenced to incarceration for two years or less. Prisons can be either state or federal facilities.

The term "correctional facilities" is rather loosely applied, but the goal at them is to rehabilitate inmates and reduce their criminal behavior, rather than simply detain them. Oakwood offers a range of rehabilitation programs aimed at preparing inmates for reintegration into society. Another goal is to reduce recidivism; that is, to reduce rearrests, reconvictions, and reincarcerations following discharge to make the community a safer place to live and work.

> ***I am not a crook.***
>
> *- Richard Nixon*
>
> ***Yeah, I'm a crook. So what?_***
>
> *- Donald Trump*

Compendium

Below is a collection of concise but detailed information and acronyms used in these Jailhouse short stories, complete with correctional terminology, housing structures, abbreviations, terms, and key elements of correctional nursing in the Oakwood jail environment.

This is provided to help readers understand the environment in which the stories take place. Jail has its own language, its own universe of codes, abbreviations, and strange customs. I created this glossary to help readers grasp the world I stepped into each day. In a way, these terms shaped every decision I made—every risk, every life saved, every mistake narrowly avoided.

Oakwood Correctional Complex

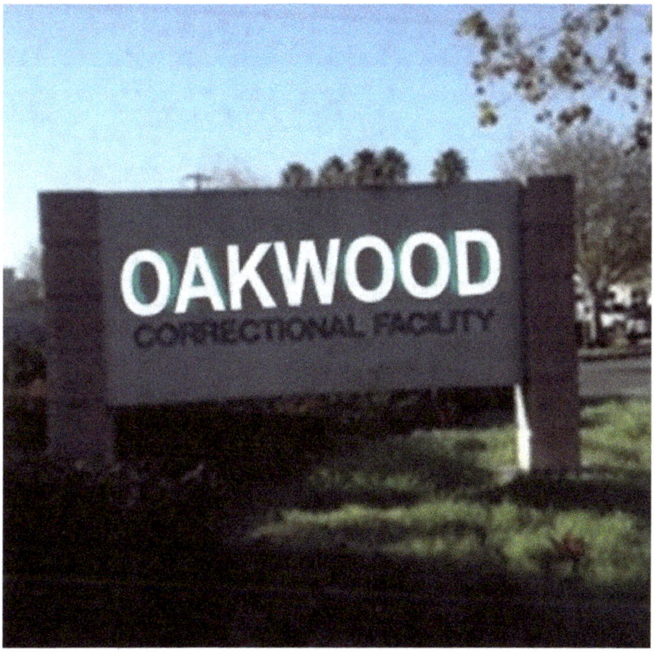

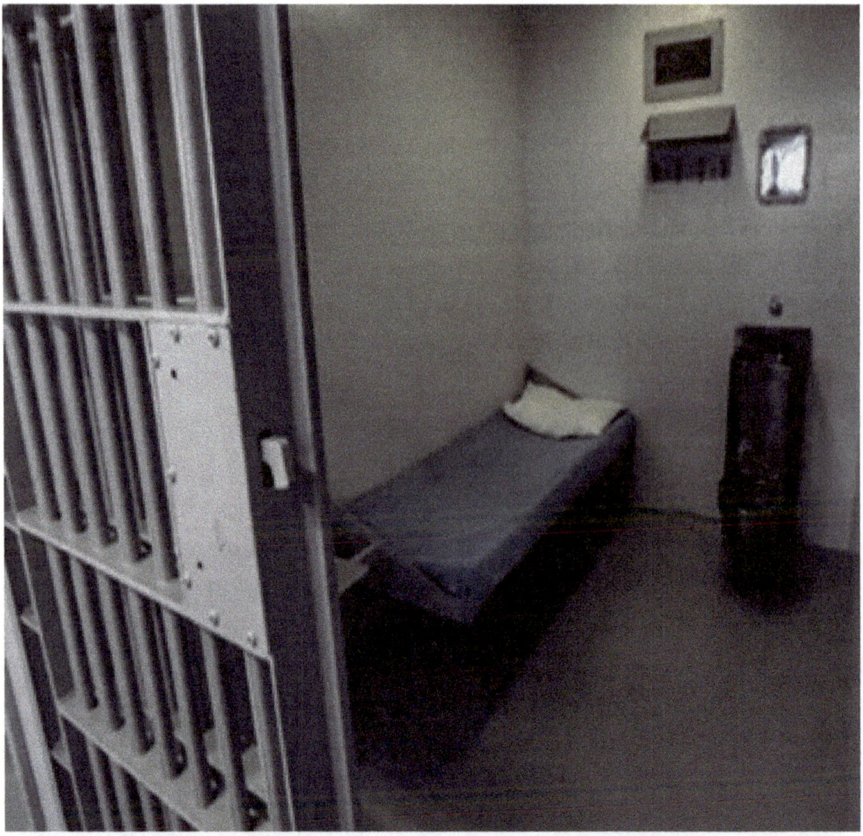

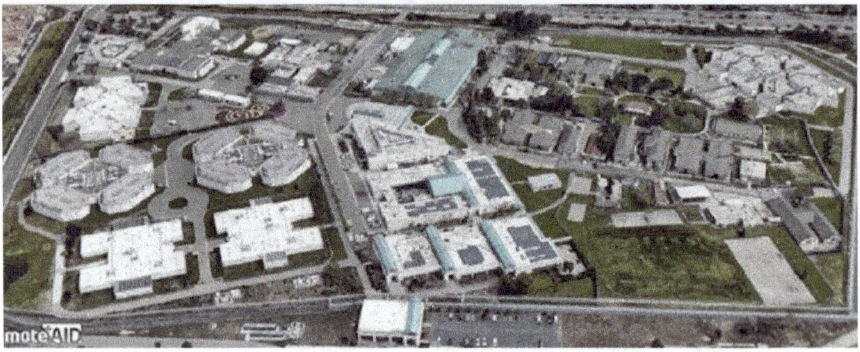

Men Care, housing, & retention of approximately 2,100 medium- and minimum-security male inmates

Camp - a military-style barracks environment for minimum security inmates

Lockdown - - buildings with medium-security cells

Women Facility houses approximately 500 female inmates, separate from the men's facility

Three levels of custody (security):minimum-, medium-,and high-security

Medical and Mental Health Services Each inmate is issued a wristband during the booking process for identification. Each inmate is interviewed at the time of booking, and a medical screening questionnaire will be completed and maintained by the Medical unit. This questionnaire is confidential and is used by the Medical staff to provide care. Answers let medical staff know if an assistive device (wheelchair or walker), accessible housing, or other help is needed while in jail. An appointment with a medical provider is made for those with disabilities. Accommodations for disability are made through the ADA Compliance unit, or by filling out a Medical Request Form (White Card) and putting it in the White Card box or giving it to a nurse at pill call. Pill calls are conducted at regularly scheduled times every day. An Officer will announce pill call in each housing area.

Each inmate is provided with a 100-page "Inmate Rulebook" and is expected to sign a form stating that they have been provided with a copy and that they must read and follow the rules in the book. The front page (signature page) is filed in the inmate's custody jacket. If an inmate refuses to sign, Witnessing Deputies write "refused."

Being incarcerated can cause a great deal of emotional stress. Inmates are advised in the Inmate's Rulebook to notify an Officer or nurse immediately if they think another inmate may be considering suicide. Some signs of stress (listed in the Rulebook) are: changes in behavior, pacing, feeling anxious, crying, writing a will, refusing medical treatment, feeling hopeless or worthless, not sleeping or eating, and looking sad or tired.

Abbreviations and Terms

ADA	Americans with Disabilities Act
ADD	Attention Deficit Disorder
ADHD	Attention Deficit Hyperactivity Disorder
ADL	Activities of Daily Living
ARMS	At-Risk Mental State
ASD	Autism Spectrum Disorder
ASL	American Sign Language
BD	Bipolar Disorder
BP	Blood Pressure
CHS	Custody Health Services (medical staff)
CN	Charge nurse is a registered nurse (RN) who oversees a nursing unit. They have advanced clinical and leadership skills that they use to supervise, delegate, coordinate, and monitor the nursing staff and patient care.
C/O	Complains of
COWS	Clinical Opiate Withdrawal Scale (protocol)Score given to patient's vital signs and symptoms (nausea, vomiting, cramps, diarrhea, difficulty sleeping) to determine the degree of opiate withdrawal they are experiencing
DOC	Department of Corrections
ER	Hospital Emergency Room
ETOH	Ethyl Alcohol (ethanol), found in alcoholic beverages, can lead to addiction and health issues
HIPAA	Health Insurance Portability and Accountability Act
IVDA	Intravenous Drug Abuse
MD	Medical Doctor
MH	Mental Health (when capitalized, refers to the Mental Health Department)
NIH	National Institute for Health
NIMH	National Institute for Mental Health
NSSP	National Strategy for Suicide Prevention
OCD	Obsessive-Compulsive Disorder
PCP	Primary Care Physician
PFN	Prisoner (or Personal) file number
PNP	Psychiatric Nurse Practitioner
PREA	Prison Rape Elimination Act - - Zero Tolerance for all forms of sexual abuse and sexual harassment
PTSD	Post-Traumatic Stress Disorder

RN	Registered Nurse
SH	Self-harm or self-harming
SMI	Serious Mental Illness

Report A record of all patients that need extra care, upcoming events for patients that require a "prep," patients having procedures that day, and all patients on detox protocols. Reports are prepared by the Charge Nurse.

White Card Medical Request Form, for help with a medical problem, mental health problem, or problem with teeth or gums; questions about medications; or to make an appointment with a doctor, dentist, or psychiatrist.

415 Code for an inmate altercation. All Deputies respond.

Lockdown Ordered confinement to a specific location, usually cells and dorms to prevent violence

5150 Refers to California law code for temporary, involuntary, psychiatric commitment of individuals who present a danger to themselves or others due to signs of mental illness. 5150 is a slang term for acting in a crazy manner.

Oakwood Medical

> *Refer to the Compendium for a brief listing of medical acronyms, abbreviations, and terms used in this book.*

Jail healthcare is like practicing medicine in a storm. People arrive detoxing, broken, terrified, and long untreated. Intake screening feels like triage on a battlefield; crises are constant. Nothing at Oakwood resembled hospital work. I learned to trust my instincts, adapt quickly, think in both clinical and security terms, and see the person beneath the charges.

A prisoner's right to medical treatment is rooted in the Eighth Amendment to the U.S. Constitution, which prohibits cruel and unusual punishment. The U.S. Supreme Court ruled in Estelle v. Gamble (1976) that deliberate indifference to serious medical needs violates the 8th amendment. Thus, correctional facilities are required to provide adequate healthcare or face constitutional claims. State laws, such as California CFR Title 15, set healthcare standards for correctional facilities, covering physician access, medication distribution, and specialized treatment.

Funding and resource allocation impact the quality of care. Affordability, staffing shortages, and treatment delays are continuing challenges. Prisoners face numerous health issues, often as a result of limited preventive care and overcrowding/understaffing. Chronic illnesses, mental health disorders, and emergency medical services are among the most pressing concerns.

Medical, dental, and mental health services are integral to the care provided at Oakwood. As mentioned, each inmate undergoes a medical screening (interview by an RN) at the time of booking. Many people arrive shattered—detoxing, broken, terrified, sick, untreated for years. Intake screening can feel like a triage battlefield; detox can feel like watching someone unravel from the inside. Information gathered is confidentially protected by the Medical unit to ensure appropriate care.

The primary Medical facility, built in the 1980s, is located close to the middle of Oakwood Correctional Facility. There is no high-tech equipment here. The Lockdown and Women's buildings are located on one side, and the "minimum camp," which houses the largest number of inmates, is on the other side of Medical.

Many inmates interact with professional staff every day; nurses and mental health staff are available 24/7. They see MDs at medical appointments, Monday through Friday. Registered nurses see inmates (patients) daily at sick call, detox checks, lab draws, diabetic call (checking blood sugar values 2-4 times/day), wound care, monitoring high blood pressure, and after "man-downs" for medical clearance. Man-downs occur surrounding altercations, accidents, ingestion of drugs, suicide attempts, hunger strikes, c/o chest pain, pregnant women in labor, and escape attempts. Inmates also have appointments with dentists, oral surgeons, orthopedic PA, psychiatrists, psychologists, and therapists in the Medical Dept.

An RN assessment after a man-down is guided by checking vital signs, dressing wounds, or calling Poison Control; all efforts are made to assess the patient's medical condition. RNs determine if the inmate needs to be sent to the ER or if they can be monitored at the facility by the nursing staff. In the event of a suicide attempt, the Mental Health staff requires that an RN clear the patient medically before the 5150 is documented. Section 5150 of the California Welfare and Institutions Code allows mental health professionals to place a person who they believe is experiencing a mental health crisis to be involuntarily detained for 72 hours when they are evaluated to be a danger to others, or to himself or herself, or gravely disabled.

Inmates know that some RNs can be fooled by a complaint of (c/o) chest pain, when the inmate wants to get sent to the ER. But the ER doctors will run basic labs and send them right back to jail. For an inmate, though, it's an opportunity to get out of jail for a little while.

Their friends will call their family after the inmate leaves the unit and is en route to the ER, hoping for a quick, very illegal visit!

On one occasion, a janitor at the ER found some duct tape hanging down from under the sink in one of the patient bathrooms. He looked closer, and it turned out to hold a huge wad of meth! The inmates would get themselves sent to the ER, ask to go to the bathroom, and bring back planted meth for their friends.

Nurses go to all buildings for pill call, diabetic checks, and to respond to emergencies. Electric golf carts are available for staff to drive to the outer buildings. Those who have time to walk can enjoy the park-like features around them: wild flowers, trees, squirrels, and birds. During evening hours, feral cats can be seen coming out to await their dinner.

Minimum-security inmates have access to medical services at the Medical Clinic. In cases of medical emergencies, inmates are instructed to notify an officer immediately. Regular pill calls are conducted, and emergency dental care can be requested. Inmates can speak with mental health staff to address any emotional stress related to incarceration, with immediate intervention available for those displaying suicidal tendencies. Patients come to Medical for diabetic checks; MD/Mental Health/Dental appointments; injuries; monitoring withdrawal from alcohol, opiates, or meth; and to sign documents (Release of Information to obtain records from pharmacies or medical records from other facilities, or permission to release medical information to family members).

Quite a few inmates with mental health diagnoses are housed at Oakwood. There are no other safe, secure facilities for these people when they get arrested. As mentioned, it has been estimated that 50% of the inmates have mental health issues. Many inmates return to custody having been off their prescribed meds for a while. These patients find that alcohol, meth, and heroin use helps to minimize their psychiatric symptoms while they are on the street. Once they are arrested and returned to jail, they must first detox from their drug of choice before a psychiatrist will restart their meds. In general, professional staff need to be more mindful when addressing this population to prevent unsafe interactions during their transition from street drugs to their prescribed medications.

The ladies' section of the jail houses up to 500 women. (In both the Lockdown dorms and the ladies' dorms of the facility, professional staff go to the specific buildings to see patients/clients where they are housed.) The ladies are classed like the men: according to charges or behavior. Once the minimum-security level men and ladies are evaluated and cleared by the Medical staff (a negative TB test, no open wounds, and no untreated medical issues) they can be given jobs as "trustees": serving meals, doing janitorial services, and doing laundry.

Medical, Mental Health, and Dental staff who decide to work in corrections experience situations unlike anything else in their careers. Patients in the hospital or in a clinic setting tend to be more compliant with their medical regimen. They are prompt in arriving at their appointments. They even have supportive family members who visit them in the hospital or take them to their clinic appointment. Professional staff working in corrections encounter patients/clients who have been off their meds for undetermined amounts of time. Some diabetics have blood sugars in the 400s with +ketones in their urine. They are having auditory and visual hallucinations. They are withdrawing from drugs and alcohol. Others are pregnant and withdrawing from heroin and alcohol. Many of the inmates know one another from the street. Coming to jail means hanging out with their friends; their friends become their family. After years of mental health issues along with drug and alcohol use, coupled with numerous incarcerations, many inmates do not have any support from their biological families. Healthcare staff who decide to work in corrections need to know their patients/clients will be completely different from anything they have ever experienced.

But people who choose to enter the health professions do so because of a desire to help people. We pursue higher education and then obtain credentials and licenses. Most of us start working in hospitals or clinics. Only after years of caring for acutely ill patients in the hospital, or at home for homecare or hospice, or following patients in a clinic, do we get the crazy idea to try working in a correctional facility. Some of us want to help this underserved portion of society. We find out rather quickly that caring for sick patients in a correctional setting is completely different from the hospital or clinic setting. Despite the fact that we are prepared with the baseline experience of caring for patients in other settings, we find ourselves overwhelmed at times while working in jail. Some medical/mental health staff do not like it because there's not enough control over the environment. For those unique individuals who choose to stay and deal with the occasional chaos and potentially dangerous situations, their lives are never the same.

Weekdays are very busy at the facility where I worked. Inmates are taken to court after breakfast; they leave for morning court at 7 a.m. The next group of inmates leaves for afternoon court after lunch, at 11 a.m. There are also specialty appointments at the local hospital, for which inmates need to be waist-chained and leg-shackled before getting in the van; they are dealing with things relating to cardiology, ophthalmology, oncology, and high-risk pregnancy. Meanwhile, there are vocational programs at the facility for inmates to participate in, learning skills to be used after release from jail: working in the kitchen, woodworking, automotive repair, landscaping, and vet technician work. Some classes enable inmates to obtain their high school diplomas. Anywhere and everywhere, deputies must pay attention at all times due to the level of (somewhat organized) chaos.

As I've shared, healthcare professionals who pursue careers in correctional settings traditionally complete their standard training in hospitals, clinics, and outpatient settings. An intriguing example comes from a conversation I had with a client during my hairdresser's appointment. She shared that she is nearing completion of her Marriage, Family, and Children's Counseling degree, which includes several weeks of direct interaction with inmates serving life sentences at a local prison. This unique experience highlights the diverse paths healthcare professionals may take in their careers, ultimately leading some to serve in facilities like Oakwood Correctional Facility, where their skills are utilized in a correctional environment.

All new employees receive orientation for their positions in the jail, which are somewhat similar to their previous positions. This process is designed to familiarize them with the unique challenges and protocols for providing medical, dental, or mental health services within a jail environment. While similarities with their prior healthcare experiences are likely, several key changes and adaptations are necessary for effective operation in this setting. For example, your patient may be in waist chains and leg shackles during the visit. You may have to wait for deputies to transport the patient to your clinic. You may have to reschedule your patient because there aren't enough deputies to transport your patient to the clinic. You may have to go to the patient's housing to complete your patient appointment. Your appointment may be interrupted by a 415, the code for an inmate altercation, to which all deputies must respond, which disrupts ongoing medical assessments and prolongs wait times.

There are time constraints for all clinics and nursing assessments. When time is up, clinic and nursing assessments are stopped as the deputies move to their next assignment. This structured timeline can be particularly challenging as it inevitably constricts the quality and continuity of care provided to inmates.

Healthcare professionals entering this environment often encounter scenarios that are vastly different from their prior experiences. The unique circumstances surrounding inmate healthcare present a range of bizarre and unexpected situations that require adaptability and quick thinking. But over time, they will learn that their role is integral to a larger care system within the correctional facility, contributing significantly to an underserved population. Understanding these dynamics is crucial for ensuring that both the health needs of inmates and the operational requirements of the facility are met effectively. Providing healthcare behind bars requires a combination of medical expertise, patience, and an awareness of the security environment.

Working in a custody setting is stressful even on a good day. Custody staff, as well as medical, mental health, kitchen, and janitorial staff, need ways to balance the stress with enjoyable, meaningful, and healthy activities. Some people play sports, go hiking, or work out at the gym.

My good friend Jelly from MH and I accidentally created an activity to help combat the impact of work-induced adrenaline on our health. It started innocently, but soon morphed into a hardcore competition...

It started with socks! I received some Christmas-themed socks as a gift and enjoyed them so much that I sent some to Jelly. She enjoyed *her* Christmas-themed socks so much that she sent me a picture of her feet with her socks on. I saw her video and felt the need to take the video up a notch. I sent her a video of my Christmas socks, the way people take videos of their kids out in the front yard! I wiggled my toes and moved the camera around for a goofy effect. After seeing my video, Jelly, being a creative, competitive sport, sent me a new video of her Christmas-themed socks in the snow on the porch of her home! Oh, it was on! My next video had my feet hanging out the window of my SUV as if they were on vacation...while parked in the driveway.

We graduated to socks with animals, flowers, and beautiful designs. I had worked in the medical field for decades; I'd begun back when nurses wore all white uniforms and their nursing caps! When I put these simple socks on before work, I found myself smiling during my shift, and thinking about the different themed socks I wore all year round; I wore Christmas socks in July! Once the videos with Jelly started, the magic of my special socks got kicked up a notch. This was years before TikTok. And over the years, the holiday-themed socks graduated to adult-themed socks that we wore hidden under our shoes. My first pair of adult-themed socks said, "WTF." Sometimes I showed the inmates my socks, and they had a good laugh, too. It was an unexpectedly effective de-stressor.

Working in a custody setting can be extremely intimidating, if not downright frightening. Chronic illness, psychiatric crises, emergency after emergency—nothing at Oakwood resembled hospital work. I had to learn to trust my instincts, move fast, adapt constantly, think in both clinical and security terms, and see the human being beneath the charges.

The deputies and officers are not only responsible for the safety of the inmates, but they are also accountable for the safety of the ancillary staff. It is an overwhelming responsibility on their part! As a nurse working in a custody setting, I was always aware of where my deputy was at all times. And for their part, the deputies were always ready to keep us safe.

My friend Jelly once relayed a very touching interaction between an officer and an inmate that gives only one example of some truly amazing people who just happen to work behind bars. A female was brought in to the booking area; she was visibly upset. The charges were horrific: first-degree murder. This was the first time this woman had been arrested. Jelly watched as one of the officers offered the woman a cup of water.

The momentary interaction demonstrated a profound experience she will never forget. As the arrestee was waiting to be booked, she exchanged a look of heartfelt gratitude with the officer as she accepted the cup of water. The officer showed a sincere but restrained look of empathy. That is the essence of my stories.

> ***You must expect great things of yourself before you can do them***
>
> - *Michael Jordan*

A Typical Day as Charge Nurse

A single shift could pull me in every direction—diabetic calls, crowded sick calls, frantic family calls, ER transfers, sudden man-downs that left my heart racing. Amid the chaos, I held onto compassion, remembering each inmate was someone's family. A quiet "thank you" or small smile often reminded me why I stayed.

It's late October, and I'm on the 3-11 PM shift, dressed in my favorite Halloween scrubs, complete with horns and a halo. I wear them proudly, and the inmates seem to appreciate my festive touch and enthusiasm for the season. My partner for the shift, nurse Skylar, is with me, ready to tackle the chaos that comes with the job.

As always, the change of each shift begins with "Report." This is, as you know, our shift change briefing, a time to catch up on everything from detoxing inmates (alcohol, opiates, benzodiazepines) to the most fragile patients: those struggling with diabetes or in immediate need of emergency care.

We get updates on the patients who were taken to the ER via patrol cars (code 1), ambulances (code 2, without lights or siren), or fire department emergency response (code 3). There's always paperwork to handle, too, including medical records from outside doctors, hospitals, and pharmacies, and Release of Information approvals to authorize us to answer requests from family members wanting to know about their loved ones locked away in jail.

Once Report is given, it's straight into the fray. The diabetic call starts, and inmates line up for their scheduled appointments with MDs, DDSs, or mental health staff. Two deputies are assigned to make sure things stay under control, keeping the medical staff safe as we work our way through the madness. It can be overwhelming when up to 40 inmates are waiting in the lobby.

Oakwood Medical's phones ring constantly. Hospital lab techs call to report dangerous lab values from the morning lab draw. Family members call in a panic for information on the status of their son/daughter. MDs call with orders, and specialty clinics call for more information on inmates they are seeing today. And that's just for starters. Staff scheduled to work later that day call in sick, and it's up to us to handle it all. Amid this chaos, each health professional must be keenly aware of their safety. Is an inmate blocking the doorway? Is an inmate close to a heavy object that could be used as a weapon?

Suddenly, the radio crackles: "Man-down: inmate on the ground, breathing, not responding, location: Main and 4th. Edward Bravo King 012." The radio transmission is repeated. The urgency of the call is clear. The radio includes the nature of the man-down as best the reporting deputy can surmise, as well as the location and the patient's record number. Main and 4th means the minimum area on the main walkway by Barracks 4. The number following it – EBK012 – is the inmate's custody ID.

The response is swift, and every unit is involved. Man-down over the radio is an instruction for all units to lock all inmates down. If an MD is in the middle of a patient appointment, it is stopped. Designated deputies from all units respond to the scene.

As Charge Nurse, I quickly assess the situation. I tell a deputy I will be responding once the inmates are locked down in the Medical lobby. The deputies get on the radio to announce who is responding to the emergency and if they are en route.

All man-downs require at least 2 RNs to respond to the event because it takes two people to carry the emergency supplies. We grab the portable crash cart loaded with IV start kits, IV solution, dressing supplies, medications used in emergencies (epinephrine, nitroglycerine, aspirin), glucometer, several oxygen tanks, AED, and a machine to take vital signs. Adrenaline pumping, I grab the laptop to access the patient's medical history. Time is of the essence.

While all this is going on, the RNs responding to the man-down still do not know the specific nature of the emergency, and are expected to walk quickly to the scene. The deputies move fast, but there are still plenty of inmates walking around in the area, and we have to keep an eye on their behavior as we make our way to the emergency. In my years at Oakwood, the inmates have always been surprisingly respectful, even helping us carry the emergency supplies up a flight of stairs when every second counts.

When we reach the inmate, it's clear that he's having a seizure. The deputies, already on high alert, call for a Code 3 Fire Department and ambulance response. The inmate, face down and seizing, is unresponsive. The nurses jump into action, laying down a clean chux pad, starting an IV, cleaning up any wounds, and preparing him for transport to the hospital.

The patient had been booked just two days before and hadn't reported any history of alcohol abuse. However, records from previous bookings show he had been treated for alcohol withdrawal. His seizures are most likely a result of that.

The Fire Department arrives quickly, administering IV Ativan to halt the seizures. As they transport the patient to the hospital, we return to the Medical unit. We make a quick call to the ER to provide a heads-up and a working diagnosis of the code 3 patient. There's no time to complete our documentation yet, but we write a quick progress note to indicate the emergency and input vital signs. The rest will have to be completed later.

We notice that many of the inmates in the lobby have left—they don't want to wait around for appointments when things take much longer than expected. The phone rings incessantly. Inmates are still waiting, and doctors try to hold appointments. The chaos never stops.

After inhaling a quick lunch, I dive back into my mountain of paperwork. Documentation from the man-down emergency takes priority, along with calling the emergency room to notify them that the patient en route has a history of ETOH abuse and seizures, and that he has an IV going.

More paperwork is needed to document phone calls or sick call slips from the inmates. Post-its are everywhere, with notes to remind me of information and details I need to record in medical charts. Patients "walk in" with complaints. If it's not an urgent medical/dental/mental health issue, the Medical deputies instruct the inmates to return the next morning to turn in a sick call slip. Sophisticated inmates know how to skip the morning sick call rush by coming to Medical after lunch to get their medical issues checked out. No line, no waiting.

The phone rang, and it was a mother worried about her son. She hadn't known where he was for days, only to discover he was in jail. Despite having a restraining order against him, she was frantic to know how he was doing. I couldn't give her any medical information, as he hadn't signed a Release of Information form. I found a note saying that he had refused to sign because he believed she was responsible for putting him in jail. She was sobbing because she was worried about his safety. I tried to comfort her by telling her that the deputies were watching over him.

I also told her I would refer him to Mental Health. He had a history of MH issues, and it didn't look like any meds had been started yet. I reassured her that the MH staff would call her after they met with him. She was crying as she hung up. I wasn't far behind.

Later, I rushed to pass this info on to my friend (and favorite Mental Health therapist), Jelly, who agreed to visit the inmate and update the mother afterward. As I headed back to the front desk, I found myself still thinking about the call, the mother's tears, and the fragile nature of the relationships we build with those behind bars.

This was a phone call I "took home" that night. Sometimes I was so touched by interactions with patients, their family, and deputies that I continued to think about them when I got home. Many things happened there at Oakwood that never happened in the hospital, hospice, or homecare setting.

By now, there is just a short time left before I need to give Report to the night shift nurses. Yet the phones continue ringing and the demands never stop. It's a never-ending cycle of phone calls, documentation, and crisis management. A single shift could stretch and twist me in every direction—diabetic call, sick call packed with pain and fear, calls from families desperate for news, ER transfers, and sudden man-down emergencies that left my heart pounding long after they ended. Amid that chaos and my need to maintain clinical focus, I tried to stay grounded in compassion, remembering always that every inmate was someone's family member. There were moments when an inmate's gratitude, or a quiet smile, or a simple "thank you" cracked me open and reminded me why I stayed. It's an exhausting job, but it's also one that reminds me of the depth of human emotion, the connections we make, and the unspoken moments that stay with you long after your shift ends.

> ***You can't do anything about the***
> ***length of your life,***
> ***but you can do something about its***
> ***width and depth.***
>
> *- Evan Esar*

Adult Custody Health Services

Building Unity Through a Multidisciplinary Task Force

Tension simmered between custody, medical, and mental health—each strained and unheard. Leadership formed a cross-department task force, bringing together staff who rarely spoke. In that room, departmental walls began to fall. We weren't departments, but people weathering the same storm. Honest conversations strengthened communication and shaped shared mission and values that improved our culture.

A few years into my work at Oakwood, I started noticing a disturbing trend. Staff complaints were increasing, and coming from every direction—physicians, nursing, medical, mental health, clerical, and even janitorial. But the real problem wasn't the complaints themselves—it was the lack of a structured way to address them. Concerns were being voiced, but no one seemed to know where to take them or who had the power to act on them.

As I sat in a leadership meeting one morning with our Medical Director, Dr. Alex Sherbakov, he looked around the room and said, "It seems like we're all hearing the same issues, but from different ends. What if we stop working in silos and come together to actually solve them?"

He had a vision: a multidisciplinary Task Force with representatives from each department and shift, designed not just to listen—but to act.

"I want real voices at the table," he said. "People who understand what it's like to walk the floor at 2 a.m., who handle intake forms, who mop the floors, who give meds under pressure. We need everyone's perspective, not just leadership." It was a bold idea. And within a month, we had our first Task Force meeting.

I remember the room that day—folding chairs in a half-circle, a whiteboard, coffee in mismatched mugs. There was Maria from night-shift nursing, Tom from janitorial, Elaine from mental health, Greg from clerical, and several others. Some people were skeptical.

"What exactly are we trying to do here?" Greg asked, arms crossed.

"We're trying to understand each other," I said. "And to fix things—together."

That broke the ice. The first few meetings were exploratory. People shared concerns from their departments, some of which had gone unheard for years.

Tom added, "I can't clean an area if I don't know it's been used. There's no communication when overtime shifts are added at the last minute." And then Greg brought up something that caught everyone off guard...

"Honestly? We don't know who half the people are walking through our area. We don't even really know who works here anymore. People start, transfer in, and disappear."

There was a pause. Then someone said, "What if we make posters? Photos, names, departments. We hang them in the breakrooms."

People nodded. "That would help a lot," Greg said.

Within two weeks, the first departmental posters went up—colorful, welcoming, with names and faces. It was a small change, but the impact was immediate. Staff began greeting each other by name. New employees felt more connected. Long-timers felt more seen. As the Task Force matured, so did our mission. One day, Dr. Sherbakov brought up a larger idea: "We've been working together to solve problems," he said. "But we don't have a shared foundation. Let's create a Vision Statement. A Mission. Core Values. Something that defines who we are as a team."

We spent weeks working through it—word by word, value by value. Respect. Accountability. Compassion. Collaboration. Partnership with our local Medical Center was central to our identity, so we made sure to highlight that as well. The final version was something we all signed—literally. Every Task Force member put their name on the document before it was framed and hung in the lobby.

<table>
<tr><th colspan="2">ADULT CUSTODY HEALTH SERVICES</th></tr>
<tr><th>MISSION</th><th>CORE VALUES</th></tr>
<tr><td>As an integral part of County Health, we work in partnership with other departments to meet the complex, challenging healthcare needs of patients residing in Adult Custody facilities, focusing on health promotion, disease prevention, and management of acute and chronic conditions.

We contribute to the general public's well-being through health education, prevention, surveillance, and treatment of communicable diseases, taking care of underserved populations and raising awareness of a variety of public health issues.</td><td>Patient care with compassion, empathy, respect, integrity, and pride

Staff: our most important resource

Teamwork: foundation of our success

Custody staff is part of our team

Streamline, re-evaluate, and continuously improve
- Work smarter, not harder</td></tr>
<tr><th colspan="2">VISION</th></tr>
<tr><td colspan="2">We operate as an integrated and empowered healthcare team by motivating, monitoring, and generously supporting one another, so that each team member reaches their full potential.

Our care exceeds regulatory and community standards, while being efficient and cost-effective. Care is rendered in a physical setting that accommodates patients' special needs.

Emphasis is on preventative care, patient education, rehabilitation, and discharge planning, which are provided with a goal of reducing recidivism.

We are nationally recognized for our excellence and leadership in the correctional health services field. We are a unique center of learning for healthcare professionals.</td></tr>
</table>

The Task Force didn't solve every problem overnight. But it changed the culture. It turned complaints into conversations. It gave everyone—no matter their role or shift—a seat at the table. And for me, it reinforced something I've come to believe deeply: when people feel heard, respected, and empowered, real change can happen.

> ***An open mind will carry you forward.***
> ***Expand your mind***
> ***and your long-term goals.***
>
> - *Quotes.com*

Diabetics in Jail

My diabetic patients became the heartbeat of my shift. At 3:30 each day, their moods reflected the jail's pulse. Some resisted, some fought, some confided—and a few even made me laugh. Even diabetic shoes became jailhouse currency. I remember Davey, who listened only when I warned him that diabetes could affect sexual function, and Mike, who kept insulin in a cooler while homeless. Their stories of addiction, heartbreak, and survival became part of my own.

The hallway outside Oakwood Medical smells faintly of bleach and musky pine-scented cleaners. It's 3:25 p.m., and the building hums with the heavy silence of a place that never really sleeps.

"Diabetics! Let's go!" a deputy calls, his voice echoing down the corridor.

One by one, men in orange jumpsuits shuffle toward the medical lobby. Some are half-awake. Others joke quietly, trying to pretend it's any other day.

At Oakwood, blood sugar checks happen twice a day—before breakfast at 3:30 a.m. and before dinner at 3:30 p.m. (Recently, breakfast was changed to 6 a.m.)

For the insulin-dependent patients, we do it again at lunch and bedtime. It's routine. Repetitive. But it's also where you really interact with people—their habits, moods, and battles all laid bare in a single drop of blood.

Years ago, the inmates did it all themselves—alcohol wipe, finger prick, test strip, insulin injection. But that ended the day one of them tried to jab a nurse with a used syringe. Nobody was hurt, but everything changed. Now, the nurses control every needle and lancet. The patients just sit, hands open, waiting.

It's a small window of time—three, maybe four minutes per person—but sometimes those few minutes stretch into something human.

Davey

I start with Davey, in his thirties, but with a boyishness about him that makes you forget his age. Brown hair always mussed, tattoos fading into old scars. His blood sugars are never good—too high, too often—but he's polite, always calling us "ma'am." He likes to tell stories that begin with, "I didn't know..."

"I didn't know my buddy's car was stolen."

"I didn't know there was a gun in the glovebox."

By now, I've heard them all.

One morning, his glucose monitor chirped out another bad number—over 250. He sighed, rubbing his temple.

"Guess I'm setting records today," he muttered.

I looked at him for a long moment. "Davey," I said, "I'm done giving you the usual lecture about your heart, your eyes, and your kidneys."

He cracked a grin. "You mean the one about how I'm gonna lose all three if I don't behave?"

"That's the one." I lowered my voice. "So let me ask you something. You plan on using *that thing* in the future?"

I pointed toward his groin.

His eyes widened. He slapped both hands protectively over himself. "Uh, yes, ma'am. Absolutely."

I leaned closer, keeping my voice just above a whisper. "Then you need to know something. High blood sugar doesn't just mess with your heart and kidneys. It damages the blood vessels *everywhere.* If you want that thing to keep working, you need to take care of yourself."

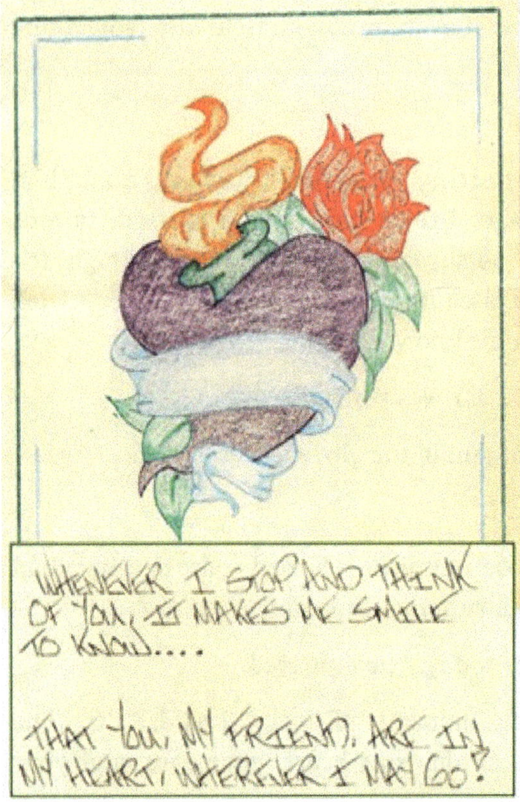

He stared at me, then broke into a nervous laugh. "You really just went there."

"I did," I said, smiling. "Because nothing else has worked."

He sat quietly for a moment, then nodded. "All right. You got my attention. Guess I'll try harder. Maybe lay off the cookies."

A week later, he slipped me a folded piece of paper during diabetic call, hiding it under a stack of forms so the deputy wouldn't see. It was a card—hand-drawn in pencil, edges smudged.

Thank you for caring, it said.

Mike

Another regular in his late forties, but who looked ten years older—thin, pale, red hair like rust under fluorescent light. The first time I met him, he smelled faintly of old smoke and rain.

He was quiet, polite, and always a little sleepy. When I pricked his finger, he'd flinch and then apologize, like pain was something he didn't have a right to feel. In the three minutes it took me to set up the glucometer, I learned more about him than I expected.

"I live in a box off El Camino," he said one night, matter-of-factly. "Got a little cooler for my insulin. Swap the ice packs out at the gas station when I can."

I stopped mid-prep. "You keep your insulin in a cooler?"

He nodded. "Gotta get creative when you're camping."

When he came in, his sugars were through the roof—200s, 300s, sometimes higher. But a few weeks inside changed him. He got some sleep. Regular meals. A steady rhythm. His sugars leveled out, his eyes cleared, and one day he showed up with a fresh haircut and a hint of pride in his voice.

"Look at me now," he said, holding out his hands. They didn't shake anymore.

When he was released that spring, I thought about driving down El Camino to see if his box was still there, maybe even say hi. But I didn't. I still wonder if he made it back to his "home."

The Shoe Game

Diabetic care at Oakwood has its quirks. The strangest one? Tennis shoes.

Because diabetics risk foot infections, they're allowed soft-sided shoes instead of the bright orange plastic flip-flops everyone else wears. Those flip-flops slap against the concrete with every step—a constant reminder that running isn't an option.

To get tennis shoes, an inmate needs a doctor's order and a custody clearance. Once approved, they get a wristband that marks them as diabetic. But inside these walls, anything of value can be traded—and those wristbands are pure gold.

It doesn't take long for the word to get around that someone's "sold" theirs.

Sooner or later, a sharp-eyed deputy spots a non-diabetic strutting around in sneakers. "Hey," he'll bark. "Medical says you're cleared for those?"

We get the call. We check the chart. The shoes and the band come off.

And the next day, the original diabetic shows up at my window. "Hey, nurse," he says, feigning innocence. "Lost my armband in a shakedown. Can I get another?"

I just smile and start the paperwork again.

Because at Oakwood, you learn two things fast—blood sugar isn't the only thing people are trying to keep under control.

Control, Care, and Trust

Working inside a jail blurs the lines between authority and compassion. Every act of care must pass through layers of security—locked doors, steel bars, deputies standing guard. Even a simple finger prick becomes a ritual of trust.

Control is everywhere. In the way syringes are counted. In the way voices echo off concrete walls. In the way a patient waits for permission just to sit down. But beneath all that control, something quieter lives—a thread of trust that we build one drop of blood at a time.

Davey trusted me enough to listen, even when I shocked him. Mike trusted me enough to tell me where he kept his insulin, out there on El Camino. And every afternoon, when diabetics file into the medical lobby, they hand me their fingers—small gestures that say, *I'll let you help me today.*

Inside these walls, control is survival. But care—that's what keeps people human.

And sometimes, when the doors slam shut behind them, and the hall goes quiet again, I think maybe that's the most important thing we do here—not just manage the numbers on a glucometer, but remind someone, even for a moment, that they're still worth caring for.

> ***Every day may not be good,***
> ***but there's something good in every day.***
> - Alice Morse Earle

No Time to Debrief

After a violent psychiatric crisis, we pulled a screaming young woman from her cell and placed her in an Observation room, where she thrashed, vomited, and gasped for air. I was shaken—but there was no time to process. Jail demanded grit and precision while my heart pounded. When it ended, we simply moved on, carrying the trauma in our scrubs. Nurses monitored continuously, with no space to recover.

I arrived at work before 3 PM, looking for Nurse Ana to give me "Report" so I could start my shift. Report showed a list of patients Ana had encountered during the Day shift who might need follow-up on 3-11 or might give me cause to expect problems during my shift.

As we talked about, sometimes patients will attempt to exhibit "symptoms" to get transported to the ER. Patients see these trips as a distraction, or a way to possibly meet up with family or a boyfriend or girlfriend. But nurses have criteria to meet before notifying the on-call MD to obtain a verbal order to transport the patient to the ER. Patients who try to see family or friends in the ER while in custody may incur more charges.

I had to meet Ana in the maximum-security unit for women, where she was responding to an ongoing man-down. These units have individual cells for inmates with serious charges, inmates who have a history of assaulting deputies, or those with difficulty getting along with other inmates. There are also inmates with serious Mental Health diagnoses on this unit. Ana was responding to the unit because of a 22-year-old female who we had had intermittently for 4 years, since the day she turned 18. The inmate had begun arguing with the deputies, and when the arguing escalated, the deputies forcibly extracted her from her cell, shackled her, and placed her in an observation room. Mental Health staff had been notified and requested to respond to the unit.

The Emergency Response Team was involved in the cell extraction. This team is composed of deputies who are specially trained for these types of emergencies, to safely move inmates to a secure location. While the inmate was shackled to the chair in the observation room she began banging her head on a table.

Mental Health staff determined the patient to be a danger to herself and promptly left the unit to write the 5150. The inmate then began to spit at the deputies and nurse, so the Emergency Response Team assembled to place the patient in a restraint chair. This chair is a last resort option, only used when all other attempts to subdue the patient have failed. (The restraint chair is a chair fastened to a base in a reclined position. The inmate is restrained there by their hands and feet.)

The encounter was turning into a psychiatric emergency!

While we were moving the patient to the restraint chair, she continued spitting at the deputies, and she began to vomit!

The spit guard mask (comprised of a veil over the top of the head and eyes, attached to a sleeve of canvas-type material over her nose, mouth, and chin) needed to be placed to avoid contamination from the patient spitting. (Note: This episode was in 2016. The face mask design has since been updated.)

Ana and I needed to remain with the patient to suction her mouth to avoid her aspirating the emesis (avoid vomit being swallowed or entering her lungs). While patients are in the restraint chair in a reclined position, RNs must monitor their vital signs every 30 minutes.

In this case, we had to monitor the patient's respiratory status as she cried and moaned like a wounded animal. Her respiratory rate exceeded 45-55/min. in her distress (normal is 16-20 breaths per minute).

Several deputies ended up nauseous and vomiting. When the inmate spat in the face of one deputy, per protocol, the deputy had to leave to be seen in Urgent Care.

This process continued for 45 minutes while Mental Health sat in their office writing up the 5150 and faxed the request to rehouse to Oakwood Control and the Acute Psych unit downtown. (In 2016 we still didn't have computers on all the units, so the documentation for the 5150 had to be written by hand.)

The patient continued to moan, cry, and hyperventilate while we all waited. After the paperwork was faxed, the ERT changed the restraint chair into a mobile device and wheeled her to the van for transport. Department Captains, Lieutenants, and the RN were present.

It was a bit shocking when the inmate's restraints were taken off...

Quietly and without difficulty, she stood up (still in waist and leg chains) and was assisted into the van. My responsibility for this patient was complete, though, I still needed to document the episode. I had a difficult night after that incident. I had to keep responding to man-downs as if nothing had happened. I had no time to debrief and recover emotionally from experiencing a psychiatric emergency. And sleep was next to impossible that night.

I was able to talk to a Mental Health co-worker the next day about how difficult the situation had been for me. I also spoke with one of the deputies who had experienced the psychiatric event; she reported having difficulty sleeping as well. My nursing co-workers were very supportive the next day. This is just one example of how the roles of RNs in a correctional facility are evolving to a daunting place. As for the deputies, they had received additional safety training as a result of an in-custody death the previous year.

After 13 years at Oakwood, this was the first psychiatric emergency I had experienced. Most other inmates who are placed in the restraint chair realize their behavior is unacceptable, and are able to calm down and come out of the chair without having to be transported to the Acute Psych Unit.

The RNs were the first responders and remained until the patient was safely transferred to the van for transport. After 13 years at Oakwood, I came to learn that there is no actual psychiatric treatment offered short of medication for patients with Mental Health diagnoses.

Since this event, Mental Health has added more clinical staff, i.e., Psychologists and specially trained therapists, who offer classes in Trauma Recovery.

> ***Keep your face towards the sunshine, and shadows will fall behind you.***
> *- Walt Whitman*

Yoda

A cheerful Vietnamese trustee became a legend for crawling through ceiling tiles—encouraged by deputies. It was equal parts absurd and unforgettable. Supervisors later discovered hidden supplies he stashed above the tiles. Despite the mischief, he was known for his spotless floors, humor, and quiet gentleness. In a heavy place, Yoda brought light, reminding me that even behind bars, joy can find a way in.

"Yoda," as he was called by the deputies (with his permission), was a likable Vietnamese male inmate in his 30s in medium-security lockdown. He was small in stature, 5'1", with somewhat large protruding ears, and an ever-present smile. He earned his nickname because of his uncanny resemblance to the famous Star Wars character.

When Yoda applied to become a "trustee," he went through the standard medical clearance process. The Medical department checked and documented his health, ensuring a current TB test and examining his arms, legs, chest, and back for any open wounds. I didn't know his real name because he took no medication nor had any treatments like wound care or blood pressure checks. Once cleared, he could be assigned regular duties. The day team has a different set of trustees and workers than the night team. Yoda was assigned to the night team.

When interviewed by the deputies, Yoda verbalized his expertise in cleaning and waxing floors. So he was allowed to wash floors every day and intermittently wax floors, which meant he had a lot of time out of his dorm. I had to admit that the floors in his unit were spotless; they sparkled under his care.

What made Yoda truly unique was his ability to move around almost unnoticed. One evening the deputies had an idea. Given his small, nimble frame, they wondered if he could navigate through the building's false ceiling. The deputies found a ladder, moved the ceiling tiles, and invited Yoda to explore. The facility consists of two large units – East and West – each with four dorms, separated by two heavy locked doors. A central Control Room, which bridged the East and West sections, controlled access.

To everyone's surprise, Yoda smoothly climbed up and crawled across the entire building with remarkable ease. The deputies considered their impromptu "experiment" a complete success.

Several weeks later, when the Sergeants discovered this unauthorized ceiling exploration, they demanded that the deputies investigate what might be hidden above those tiles. They found that Yoda had secretly stashed cleaning and buffing pad supplies in his hidden sanctuary. No one ever caught Yoda up in the ceiling again, making this a legendary one-time adventure.

His legacy? Perfectly waxed floors and a legendary tale of a small man who found the most creative storage solution imaginable – right above everyone's heads!

> ***Success is a journey, not a destination.***
> ***Just keep learning and keep growing.***
> *@Inspirehard*

Heroin Withdrawal in Jail

Withdrawal strips people raw—trembling bodies, erupting skin, unraveling minds. Yet even in dark moments, I saw striking humanity: Cody, who explained biologics better than some clinicians, and Jolly Jon, who laughed through abscess pain that would break most people. They reminded me addiction isn't identity—it's a battle often fought alone.

Before working at Oakwood, I had never worked with patients who were detoxing. The subject of detox was not even addressed in nursing school. When I started at Oakwood, I initially learned that withdrawing from alcohol and benzos can be life-threatening without medical supervision.

Eventually, nurses were given protocols to monitor patients, complete with reports of daily opiates use during the booking process. My assignments included assessing patients who were detoxing from these addictive substances almost every shift. I observed that patients withdrawing from heroin (an opiate) were, as a group, quiet, respectful, and suffering in silence.

When someone is arrested, a portion of the booking process involves evaluation by an RN. Every inmate must be medically stable to be housed at Oakwood.

Wounds, unstable blood sugar, elevated blood pressure, or any injuries from a car accident or a dog bite need to be medically cleared in our contracted ER before inmates can be housed in jail.

Among the questions every person being booked is asked: "Are you currently using medication that could cause withdrawal symptoms?"

Sometimes the person tries to hide drug or alcohol use, only to experience severe withdrawal symptoms 2-3 days later. Withdrawal from alcohol and benzos without medical support can be life-threatening. But inmates who are ashamed of their drug use or who truly believe they will be bailed out before they feel sick may deny using.

A couple of inmates who were withdrawing from heroin made a big impression on me.

Cody, a 30-year-old heroin addict, came to Medical for an assessment of his withdrawal.

Our protocol is called the Clinical Opiate Withdrawal Scale (COWS). The patient's vital signs are checked, and they are asked if they are experiencing nausea, vomiting, stomach cramps, diarrhea, etc. A score is given to determine the degree of withdrawal they are currently experiencing.

Cody looked 10 years older than his stated age. He appeared somewhat unkempt, with areas of flaking skin on his face. He had several small open wounds on his face and several days of beard growth. I checked his vital signs, and they were stable. He commented that he was having difficulty sleeping, which is one of the symptoms associated with heroin withdrawal.

His primary complaint during the assessment was persistent itching of rashes on his arms, legs, chest, and back.

Upon closer inspection, I saw that he was covered with a thick, flaking rash. When inmates come to Medical, they are expected to be dressed appropriately. This was wintertime. But inmates must take off their jackets in the lobby before entering the Medical office...

Cody had on a long-sleeved thermal top, so I needed to take him to the treatment room and secure a screen to check his arms, legs, chest, and back for psoriasis. Both arms, both legs, his chest, and his back were affected. I offered him our Standardized Procedure for rashes: Benadryl, 50 mg, 3 times a day for the itch as needed orally, and a topical cream with a steroid in it.

He was very polite and said, “Thank you," and left. He then returned the next day for an assessment of his opiate withdrawal. (Unbeknownst to me, another nurse had requested a “welfare check” for his chronic skin condition).

As I began my assessment of Cody, I asked him if he had followed up with an MD or Dermatologist for his psoriasis. He replied he had an MD and a Dermatologist who both agreed he had the worst case of psoriasis they had ever seen. I asked him if he had ever tried the most advanced treatments for psoriasis, which are injections that interfere with the cycle of the plaques involved in the disease.

Cody looked up and said, "I have held off on trying Biologics as each generation seems to be followed by patients who are involved in class action lawsuits because of the side effects from these medications. I'm waiting for a more reliable Biologic to start treatment."

I admit that hearing these specific details about pharmaceuticals from a heroin addict covered in itchy psoriasis stopped me cold. Cody spoke with such insight and intelligence regarding the pharmaceutical industry!

It was a humble reminder to remember that there is a human being under the façade of drug addiction. Good Luck Cody!

***

Jon is a 39-year-old man in Medium-security lockdown housing, who admitted to the Booking nurse that he would need medical support for heroin withdrawal. He expressed frustration because he had just been released five days previously, and was already back in jail. The nurses were checking him for alcohol and heroin withdrawal.

Heroin addicts have admitted to me that they will state alcohol abuse in addition to heroin because they will be guaranteed detox meds around the clock, not just “as needed” for heroin withdrawal.

“Jolly Jon” had a big smile on his face, and he spoke to the nurses and officers in a very respectful manner. He was 6'3" and well built; his lifetime of intravenous drug abuse and alcohol did not manifest in his build. The only obvious signs were under his clothing: abscesses on his bilateral upper arms and bilateral lower legs. He kindly signed a refusal for assessment of his alcohol withdrawal and wounds, but took his Librium and antibiotics.

After 3 days, he came up to me and said, "These abscesses are really starting to hurt." His temperature was 102.9F. I was concerned he might be septic from his years of intravenous drug abuse (IVDA). He was still friendly and joking, but it was obvious he didn't feel good. I called the MD on-call and got an order to send him to the ER. I was grateful he agreed to go.

I saw him two days later, after a couple of days off. He sounded like his old jolly self. He pulled out all the wound packing from the abscesses and refused all wound care. Jon claimed he felt better without the packing. And he thanked me for sending him to the ER. He said he had all the ER staff laughing while he was there. I believed him.

It concerned me that he had signed a refusal for wound care. Abscesses that are not properly dressed can recur. In any case, he was released two days later.

I will always remember Jolly Jon as a friendly, joking, respectful, and kind patient, who happened to be a heroin addict. These men reminded me that addiction is not identity; it is a battle—one many are fighting alone. I wondered sometime later if incarceration may have saved his life, for a little while at least.

> ***It is never too late to be***
> ***what you might have been.***
> *-George Eliot*

Compassionate Release

I once advocated for a man to get early release so he could care for his dying mother, believing I was helping a family heal. When I learned he'd stolen her morphine so he could sell it, disappointment hit me like a punch to the gut. It taught me that compassion is never guaranteed to land where you hope, even when intentions seem pure —but it's still worth offering.

One particularly memorable interaction involved an inmate whose mother was dying. During a routine wound dressing, he shared his deep worry about her condition. Learning that she was with the same hospice where I'd worked for many years, I was motivated to help.

"How long is your jail sentence?" I asked him.

"Several more months," he responded.

My mind started going crazy, trying to think of a way to get him released to help out his mother before she passed away. I called hospice the next day and explained this young man's situation to one of the supervisors. "I may be able to arrange for a compassionate release for the inmate to provide care to his terminally ill mother," she offered.

I gave the supervisor the inmate's name, the mother's name, and her location. The supervisor confirmed that the inmate's mother was currently on service with hospice. The supervisor then notified the hospice chaplain, who coordinated with the Oakwood chaplain. They exchanged information, and the process toward the compassionate release began. These are rarely approved.

Two weeks later, the inmate was released a couple of weeks earlier than his scheduled date. He went to his mother's home to learn about how he could provide her with the best possible care for her terminal condition.

The story took an unexpected turn, though. A couple of weeks later, I called to find out how he was doing, caring for his mother. I spoke with the supervisor who had helped organize the release. She laughed and laughed and laughed! Hospice work can be very challenging. Laughing (and crying) is important for people working in this field. The supervisor then took a long breath.

“Well, it started out really good,” she said. “The son was there to help his dying mother. BUT.....he eventually took her liquid morphine and sold it for cash!"

It is exceedingly rare for caregivers to commit this kind of illegal act.

Hospice administrators demanded that the son be removed from the home or she would lose her hospice services. “I don’t want my son to leave!” the mother demanded. So, our hospice discharged her from service. But she was able to obtain hospice services from a different agency.

> ***Life is too short to wake up with regrets.***
> ***So love the people who treat you right.***
> ***Forget about those who don’t believe.***
> ***Everything happens for a reason.***
> ***If you get a chance, take it.***
> ***If it changes your life, let it.***
> ***Nobody said life would be easy.***
> ***They just promised it would be worth it.***
>
> *Quotesgram.com*
> *- inspirational quotes about life*

Fantasy Wedding

Catherine, a mentally ill and unhoused woman, endlessly spun dazzling fantasies of her own wedding—celebrities attending, gowns sketched in vibrant color, plans for a life she'd never touch. Her imagination floated through the dorm like glitter. Even though her delusions were anchored in trauma, they gave her—and all of us—a reprieve from the heaviness around us. She reminded me that dreams can survive even in confinement.

Working at Oakwood Correctional Facility has been an adventure, especially in the maximum-security women's building. We've got two distinct dorms here. One dorm houses women with mental health challenges who struggle to get along. Many here have a history of assaulting deputies. The other has women facing serious charges. Some of these ladies are in custody for extended periods, and I get to know them better than those who pass through quickly.

It is fascinating to witness their transformations. From the moment of their arrest to getting their medications restarted, some of these women undergo incredible changes. The psychiatric process is complex. Doctors fax prescriptions for inmates with mental health diagnoses, but tragically, many never pick up their medications after release. Instead, they often turn to drugs and alcohol. If they are rearrested, they must go through detox before psychiatrists will start their meds.

A particularly touching story that's stayed with me involves Catherine. At 57, she'd been in and out of jail for years, unhoused, with untreated mental and medical issues. Her family had filed a restraining order against her. Despite her challenges, she was always cheerful and friendly. I was distributing medications one evening when I heard her excited voice: "Nurse Nancy, I'm getting married!"

I looked towards where the voice originated and saw Catherine waving and smiling. She had been in jail for six weeks and was not taking her medical or MH meds. She was so excited. "Nick and I are getting married at the beach in Santa Cruz." Carlos Santana had supposedly been hired to perform at the reception.

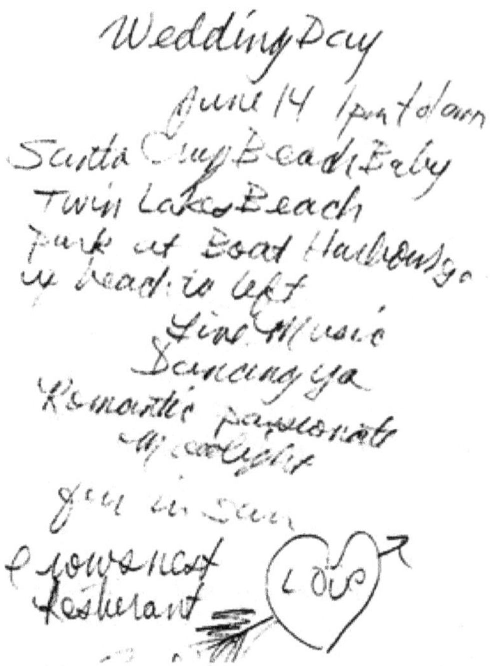

Catherine's wedding invitations had become legendary. She would draw them out by hand, complete with highlights of the event. When incarceration interfered, her wedding plans would simply be rescheduled, and she would write new invitations. Several custody staff members and I received many handwritten "wedding invitations" over the years. She became one of my favorite inmates. I haven't seen her in years. But I genuinely hope she's doing okay living on the streets.

My experiences at Oakwood have taught me that humanity exists in the most unexpected places. Whether caring for patients, supporting inmates through medical challenges, or simply listening, there are moments of profound connection everywhere.

The facility might seem intimidating from the outside, but inside, it's a microcosm of human stories; of struggle, hope, failure, and occasional triumph. I got enjoyment from bettering the essence of humanity, and I'm grateful to be a small part of these stories.

> ***Nothing is impossible.***
> ***The word itself says 'I'M POSSIBLE'***
> *- Audrey Hepburn*

Home Away from Home

Oakwood's second floor, designed to be an infirmary, became overflow housing during repairs—a strange social experiment. Mentally unstable women flooded plumbing by flushing sheets in toilets; protective-custody inmates scrubbed floors spotless, then tried to take apart the recreation deck out of boredom. Their reactions revealed both resilience and unpredictability—and how jail operations must constantly adapt.

When the building at Oakwood, which houses Medical, Mental Health (MH), clerical, and janitorial staff, was being planned, the idea was for the second floor to serve as an infirmary for Medical and offices for Custody. The layout was all set: a nursing station, isolation cells for maximum-security or seriously ill inmates, and several cells with four bunk beds. There were even showers down the hall for the inmates to use.

But when the building was finally completed, there weren't enough nurses to staff the infirmary. So instead of the building being used for its original purpose, medical patients from Oakwood were sent to the Main Jail for care, and the second floor ended up as offices for Custody and storage for medical supplies.

Over time, the older buildings at Oakwood started to show their age—things like plumbing, electrical systems, heating, cooling, and even paint were all breaking down. That's when the second floor got a new purpose: temporary housing for dorms undergoing repairs.

Now, depending on which group of inmates was being moved upstairs, Medical and MH staff downstairs saw changes in how they went about their day.

The first group that moved upstairs were female inmates with MH diagnoses. If the women were stable enough to be in a group setting—meaning they could interact without causing harm—they were placed in the rooms with four bunks. Inmates who had difficulty interacting with other inmates got a single cell.

Sometimes, the women had difficulty keeping up with self-care, such as daily showering, though the other inmates in their dorm were generally understanding. Being incarcerated is tough, and for some, it was even harder. Everyone knew the rules, and if you didn't follow them, you would get "locked down" longer as punishment.

In an attempt to obtain more time outside their cells, a few women would attempt to flush things like sheets down the industrial-strength toilet. This, of course, caused major plumbing problems. The toilets would overflow, making the cells unusable.

But the bigger issue happened downstairs. Sewage would literally start dripping through the pharmacy ceiling, forming foul-smelling puddles of amber liquid on the floor. Keep in mind that there was only one pharmacy, and the nurses had to walk in and out of it all day. Thankfully, the facility's plumbing staff addressed the problem quickly.

A few years ago, a deputy discovered something alarming in a Protected Custody building. Inmates in one of the dorms had managed to create a hole in the wall that led to the outside. This opening wasn't visible on any of the cameras. But it was accessible to the trustees on the landscaping team and also to visitors to the building. The deputies had no idea how long it had been there.

Once the hole was discovered, all the dorm's inmates had to be moved upstairs to the second floor while repairs were made. Now, this group of inmates was *completely different* from the female inmates with MH diagnoses. Many of them were gang-affiliated, and gang rules were strict. One of the big rules? Keep your cell clean and orderly. The idea of intentionally overflowing a toilet was completely unacceptable. Needless to say, plumbing issues weren't a problem when it came to this group.

Part of the plan to house inmates on this floor included allowing them to go outside. To make that possible, a small fenced area, kind of like a box, was added to the 2nd floor. This allowed them to get fresh air at scheduled times during the day, as mandated by law. But it only took a couple of days for deputies to realize that the inmates were slowly dismantling the outside fenced area. Officers found missing nuts and bolts among the inmate's belongings.

A team of engineers had to be brought in to repair the deck to make it safe for future inmates.

> ***In three words, I can sum up everything I've learned about life: it goes on.***
>
> *- Robert Frost*

Rose

During a chaotic shift, Rose, a mentally ill woman, visibly unraveling, began crying out, "Call 9-1-1." Mental Health missed the seriousness of her condition until a seasoned therapist recognized acute schizophrenia requiring emergency care. As deputies calmed her by softly singing spirituals, the unit shifted—crisis giving way to an unexpected moment of tenderness and compassion.

Tuesday afternoon started like a typical weekday at Oakwood. As Charge Nurse on the day before a full moon, I was ready for the wacky, wild, and unexpected things that always happen for the "Full Moon Extravaganza!"

From my experience in numerous jobs in hospitals, home care, and hospice, there were always full-moon experiences among patients. Ask any nurse.

I got a call at 3 PM from a deputy sheriff in the Level 4 women's dorm. These were the ladies who had difficulty interacting with others because of mental health issues, or were just generally unhappy people, so they were isolated in single cells. The deputy called to report that one of the ladies had fallen and needed a nurse to come and assess her injuries.

3 PM marks the change of shift, which means that the exhausted day-shift nurses needed to respond. Meanwhile, the PM shift nurses were preparing to begin their shift. If it is a serious call, both the Day and PM shift nurses must respond. The Day shift nurse went out to the dorm. I was receiving the Report: a record of all patients that needed extra care, any upcoming events for patients that required a "prep," patients having procedures that day, and all the patients on detox protocols. The Day-shift Charge Nurse identifies all significant patient events during the day. It usually takes 30 minutes to finish the Report.

The day shift nurse called from the patient's dorm to report that the patient who had fallen was Rose, a 44-year-old African-American woman. Rose had been hospitalized for hypertension two days after her arrest. Before her fall, many staff members had interacted with her. Now Rose had fallen and injured her right shoulder. The nurse brought her to Medical for further assessment. Rose had been hospitalized for a week for her blood pressure to regulate. After hospitalization, she was housed in the women's medical unit for close observation. She was eventually rehoused in the Level 4 unit, where inmates who have difficulty getting along with others are placed.

One morning, Rose went to court. In the courtroom, she complained of chest pain and was taken to Stanford Hospital, where she spent the night. She was medically cleared and returned to Oakwood the following day. The Charge Nurse assessed Rose when she arrived at Oakwood and determined she was stable enough to return to level 4 housing.

When Rose arrived at Oakwood Medical, I spoke with her. Her BP was dangerously high. The day shift nurse had called the on-call MD for further orders for care. I explained to Rose that I needed her to sign a Release of Information to authorize Stanford to provide their records of her hospital stay, including labs performed, meds given, and schedule of any follow-up appointments.

Rose was quite agitated; she kept yelling, "Call 9-1-1, Call 9-1-1".

She was crying and asking me to read the form to her. Rose also seemed somewhat mentally altered, and I couldn't figure out what was going on. She'd had the two previous inpatient hospitalizations at two different hospitals. She'd also been seen in Booking and medically and mentally assessed by RNs at her arrest and after each hospitalization.

The only diagnoses in her medical record were hypertension and a history of depression. The Day shift nurse spoke with the on-call MD about her shoulder injury and obtained a verbal order for an X-ray of her shoulder and Motrin for pain as needed. She had already hung up before I told her about Rose's altered mental status.

I was desperate.

I hand-wrote a referral to Mental Health for her persistent crying and her history of depression and hand-carried it to the Mental Health office (this was back in the day when we had hybrid medical records).

I pleaded with everyone in the office to help me with Rose.

Judy stepped up and said, "I walked over with Rose when she was brought to Medical."

Judy also indicated that she had just gotten off the phone with Rose's aunt, who was very worried about her niece.

I explained that Rose had been brought to Medical for a possible shoulder injury, but began crying and yelling to call 9-1-1. Rose's mental status was in question.

In a calm voice, Judy offered to see Rose. After Rose spoke with Judy for a few minutes, Judy stuck her head out of the exam room and asked,

"Is Rose on her psych meds?"

I looked at her for one second and slowly shook my head no.

Judy had a look of terror on her face.

Judy came back to me and reported, "Rose is schizophrenic and needs her meds!"

Then Judy immediately wrote up a 5150 for transfer to the Acute Psych Unit downtown.

I asked Judy, "How could the many, many professionals who saw her have missed this diagnosis?"

Looking back, this may have been the beginning of the great work relationship I ended up having with Judy.

As Judy finished her paperwork, I sat with Rose, who was convinced the deputies wanted to kill her. Rose asked for a telephone so she could say goodbye to her family.

Just then, Deputy Benson walked in. The Medical deputies were all male. Any time there is a female inmate in Medical, a female deputy must stand by. So I explained the situation to Deputy Benson, a gorgeous African-American woman.

Deputy Benson began speaking to Rose calmly.

Then after a few minutes, Rose started singing in the most beautiful voice!

Moments later, Deputy Abbott (another beautiful African-American woman) from Classification came to Medical – she was there to evaluate Rose and reclassify her to go into Mental Health housing.

Deputy Abbott joined Deputy Benson and Rose, and soon the three of them could be heard singing what the deputies referred to as "Negro spirituals" together! As the deputies calmed her, their voices softened the air for everyone, creating a rare moment of beauty and tenderness. I felt compassion blooming in crisis. These deputies had completely cheered up Rose and put her in a wonderful state of mind with song.

When I thought about the synchronicity of this situation, I smiled. It had begun one way and then transformed into something else entirely!

Full Moon Extravaganza!

> ***Every day is a new beginning.***
> ***Take a deep breath, smile, and start again.***
> *- author unknown*

Leaving A Mark

Inmates live by codes few outsiders understand: share emergency contacts and never pursue another's partner. When one man broke that rule, the slash across his face was swift and brutal. While deputies searched for the weapon, I cleaned and closed the wound, struck by how survival shapes inmate justice. That scar would follow him forever, a permanent mark and warning etched into skin.

There are commonly accepted "rules" among inmates that are understood by most of those who come and go to and from jail. One of the accepted "rules" is that you always give your emergency phone number and contact person info to your fellow inmates; this is in case of an emergency, and/or if the inmate cannot contact their family. If the inmate can't call, their buddies will call the family to let them know they are on their way to the hospital, with details of what occurred to warrant the trip. But if the family does show up at the hospital, they are at risk of being arrested, as the inmate is not allowed visitors in the ER. The staff usually finds these things out accidentally, when inmates talk with nurses they trust.

Another "rule" among inmates is that guys don't go out with inmates' girlfriends or wives when they are in jail. When that happens, the incarcerated man will inevitably find out. They always find out. But the jilted inmate can't retaliate in any way while in jail. All bets are off, however, if the guy who dated an inmate's lady gets arrested and comes to jail. Somehow, the guy who broke the rule always ends up in the same dorm as the betrayed inmate. When this happens, the custody staff and the nurses end up getting involved.

The nurses were called to a lockdown dorm after two inmates attacked another inmate. In addition to bumps and bruises, the right side of his face was slashed from the ear to the jaw with a homemade shank. Copious amounts of blood were gushing from the wound. He was drenched in blood and a pool was forming on the ground. Nurses responded to the man down. Code 3 was called (fire department, complete with lights, sirens, and an ambulance). Dressings were applied in an attempt to stop the bleeding.

Sometimes a wound on the side of the face doesn't stop at the jaw; it continues to the neck, close to the carotid artery. Vital signs are assessed, neuro checks are done to assess if the person incurred a head injury during the altercation, and he is handed over to the Fire Department and ambulance personnel for transport to the ER. Occasionally, the inmates are released to jail with 30-40 sutures to close the wound. Other times, the injuries are so severe that they end up in ICU. Once the wound heals, there is a lasting reminder on their face to themselves and all others who understand the "rule": that this person broke the "rule" and the appropriate penalty was administered.

This is a terrifying sight to an untrained nurse. When it happens, Medical (the nurses) come in and take over, and the inmate is transported to the ER. After the inmate leaves, Hazmat cleans up all the blood. Then, and only then, do the deputies investigate the altercation. Deputies conduct Interviews to determine which inmates participated in the dispute.

At some point, the dorm has a "shakedown" so staff can look for the weapon. The weapons aren't always found and confiscated. This is a major concern to Medical and Mental Health staff who see inmates in the dorm. The deputies do their best to keep themselves and civilian staff safe, but they can't always find all weapons. This is one story that reveals the unspoken codes by which inmate culture enforces its own justice.

> ***No pressure, no diamonds***
>
> *- Thomas Carlyle*

Parking Lot Adventures

Late shifts meant walking to my car beside newly released inmates. One woman serenaded the parking lot, certain she was the next Mariah Carey. Another night, a lost elderly man circled in fear until a deputy found a taxi for him. But the night a recently released man approached me in the dark—my pulse roaring—changed everything.

I worked 3-11:30 PM for most of my career at Oakwood. Nurses, mental health staff, and clerks would finish our tasks (on a good night) around 11:15 PM, and put things away in anticipation of leaving at 11:30 PM. One significant problem with leaving work from a correctional facility versus a hospital at midnight is that inmates are also being released at that time. We all pass through the same door, the West Gate. The deputy in charge will usually give us a heads-up if a group of inmates has been recently released. They could be waiting in the parking lot to be picked up by a family member, or just hanging out. One time, an inmate released at night promptly broke into one of the employees' cars. He was quickly rearrested.

One evening after midnight, I walked out to the parking lot with Nancy, who works for the Department of Corrections (DOC). She issues inmates clothes to change into when they arrive at Oakwood and returns their clothes to them when they are released.

We were both part of the small group of volunteer staff who take care of the feral cats who live at Oakwood. That night, we had already fed the cats. We were headed out to get a trap to try to catch two older cats who were getting quite thin and needed to retire.

A young woman in her 20s approached us. She had her purse and held some keys in her hand. She stopped and said, "Can you help me?"

We turned to her and answered, “Yes,” thinking she may need directions.

She said, “My name is Melissa. I need to find my car. I can't find my car.” We asked her if she had just been released from Oakwood. She replied, “Yes, and I can't find my car.”

We said to her, “But if you got arrested, your car wouldn't be here.” Then: “Do you have family to call? Where are you going?” Melissa replied, “I'm married. My husband and I live in Monte Sereno. I'm the next Mariah Carey.” She then sang to us in the parking lot to show off her melodious voice.

At that point, we realized Melissa probably had some Mental Health (MH) issues. She didn't seem to understand what we were talking about. We were also worried about her safety. We gently suggested that we all return to the West Gate, where all staff and inmates leave. We assured her we could get some help from the Oakwood deputy who supervised the entrance.

We entered through the door together. Melissa walked along with us, rambling about being the next Mariah Carey and finding her husband. We approached Deputy Small, a seasoned deputy. We said, “Deputy Small, we met Melissa in the parking lot. She told us she lives in Monte Sereno. She is looking for her car in this parking lot. She is the next Mariah Carey. Can you help get her home safely?” We were hoping our description of Melissa would imply that she had MH issues and needed support.

Deputy Small replied, “Miss Melissa, I told you to go catch the bus! Now GO GET ON THE BUS!”

Melissa quietly replied, “Okay.”

Nancy and I stared at each other in total disbelief! This deputy was not willing to help this poor woman by calling his Sergeant to request a courtesy drop-off at the hospital, with whom we have a contract to care for inmates. We had Sergeants approve drop-offs for other at-risk inmates at the hospital who weren't safe on their own when they were released. Melissa was probably a “new” booking, arrested the day before. MH could have arranged a taxi if they had met with her and determined she wasn't safe on her own. But we didn't question his decision. He could have made a lot of trouble for Nancy and me. We sadly watched Melissa walk out the door. And we prayed that she would safely arrive at her home that night.

The next parking lot story has a better ending. A year later, working in Oakwood Medical, I saw Helen, one of the best MH staff. I was Charge Nurse and met her in Medical at the front desk. She let me know she was expecting a 74-year-old gentleman referred to her following his appearance in court; he had displayed confusion. The older man couldn't remember that he had been to court earlier that same day. Helen was concerned for his safety in his current housing: a barracks with 60 men of all ages, with minimal supervision.

She began to make notifications to rehouse him to another facility where he could be more closely supervised. Then Helen found out the inmate was being released. She re-interviewed him to determine if someone could come pick him up and give him a ride home upon his release. He assured her he would call his girlfriend for a ride. The inmate left to be processed for release.

Later that same night, I walked out at the same time as Helen. We were both leaving long after all the other staff had left, so we were alone in the parking lot after midnight. We noticed an older man wandering around out there. Helen recognized him as the same man she had spoken to earlier, who had assured her his girlfriend would come pick him up.

We went to him. Helen asked him if he had called his girlfriend. He replied, "I don't have her number after all. Things are missing from my wallet."

His cell phone was at his residence, 20 miles away. The man asked if someone could point him to a motel, so he could make other arrangements in the morning.

Helen and I brought him back to West Gate, where Deputy Richards was working the area. Helen explained that the man was confused and had no ride home. The deputy looked in the man's wallet and found a credit card. He called for a taxi. Deputy Richards then pulled up the address on his court papers and confirmed it with the man. He also copied down the cell phone number. The deputy safely helped the man get in the taxi and gave the driver the correct address.

Two hours later, Deputy Richards called the cell and the man answered. He had made it home safely. The man's only concern was locating his girlfriend. Deputy Richards said he couldn't help him there.

Because of the few extra minutes Deputy Richards had taken to arrange for a ride and follow up with a call, this man made it home safely. Helen and I both sent letters of commendation to his superiors.

One summer evening, a rooster appeared at the south end of the employee parking lot! It appeared to be missing tail feathers, but was getting around okay. It pushed the two feral cats in the parking lot out of the way to eat some of their kibble. Once word got out about a rooster in the parking lot, several employees brought food for the rooster. With its own food, it stayed away from the cats.

Attempts were made to find a rescue to come pick it up. It slept on the hood of the service vehicles parked at the south end of the lot. At 3 am, it began crowing, which was how we had determined it to be a rooster. Inmates in the minimum camp barracks heard it. It crowed until the morning! Much to the surprise of the Oakwood staff, none of the inmates complained about the crowing! This was an unexpected surprise, coming from the middle of a bustling metropolitan area. Maybe it was a reminder of simpler times. The rooster eventually found a forever home with one of the deputies.

One night after I'd retired, I volunteered to feed the feral cats at Oakwood. I had been feeding them for nine years while I was working, and for three years since I retired. When working, I would feed the cats living on the grounds inside the jail first. When I left the facility, I would drive to the end of the parking lot and feed the two cats that lived outside the security fence.

Now that I am retired, when I arrive to feed the cats around 10 PM, I start in the parking lot.

This happened to be a busy weeknight; there were plenty of cars in the parking lot, not only staff vehicles, but also visitors' vehicles. I drove down to the end of the lot, put my car in Park, grabbed food and water, and left my car running with the door open because it only takes three minutes to feed, water, and say, "Hi," to the cats. Then I'm back in my car to park and go feed the cats living inside the Oakwood facility. This is what I have done for the three years since I retired.

This particular night, I drove to the area where I feed the "parking lot" cats. No cameras, no staff patrolling the parking lot. I pulled around, stopped, placed my car in Park, left the car running (it is a hybrid, so sometimes it sounds off when it's on), and got out to feed the cats who were waiting for me.

While I am finishing up, a tall young man walks up to me and asks, "How do I get out of here? I need to catch the bus."

I was shocked; this guy had just been released from Oakwood, and I'd missed seeing him walking around the parking lot! I was completely caught off guard.

I explained that there is a fence around the facility, and he would need to walk back the way he came to find the exit. Standing next to my car, he asked, "Whose car is this? Can you give me a ride?"

I quickly said, "It's my car. I'm going to work after I feed the cats."

He bought my story and turned around and left. I was still shaking when I got back in the car. I slowly drove to park so I could go inside and feed all the other cats. When I walked into the West Gate, he was sitting in the visitors' waiting area!

I quietly told the deputy what had happened in the parking lot; he said he would keep an eye on him. I got my visitor's badge and went in to feed the cats. I came back 15 minutes later, and he was gone. He'd taken off after I went in to feed the cats. The deputy asked if I would like an escort to my car. I declined the offer. As I walked to my car, I scanned the parking lot.

After all the "Safety Classes" I had sat through every two years at Oakwood, I'd found myself in a potentially unsafe situation, with no one around, and out of the range of the cameras. Now, whenever I pull up in the parking lot to feed the cats (scanning the area as I drive), I park my car at the end of the parking lot, turn off the engine, grab the food and water, get out, and lock my vehicle!

Every Time.

> ***Life is 10% what happens to you***
> ***and 90% how you react to it.***
> *- Charles R. Swindoll*

Eliann

The night Eliann, severely mentally ill, plucked out her own eye will never leave me. She murmured scripture as blood pooled and deputies shouted; my hands were shaking as I tried to stabilize her. Afterward, I felt hollow and couldn't sleep, returning to Mental Health, desperate to unload what I'd seen. The trauma scarred us all; I eventually sought psychiatric support. Some experiences don't fade—they burrow in.

It amazes me how the Universe sometimes picks a special group to witness something mind-blowing. It's like we're randomly selected for an incredible, jaw-dropping moment that totally challenges everything we thought we knew. Together, we stand in shared amazement, trying to process the unbelievable and find words to capture an experience that defies explanation. This was one of those moments.

It was Friday afternoon, 3:15 p.m. The PM shift was listening to Report from the Day shift and preparing for their assignments.

The radio snapped to life: "A nurse is needed immediately in the Women's Special Management dorm. One of the inmates has popped her eye out!"

We stared at each other, trying to absorb what we had just heard. The words were so unexpected that they were beyond comprehension.

Women's Special Management – a mental health dorm – is the one to which I was assigned. I knew I needed to get to the dorm IMMEDIATELY. As I rushed toward the dorm, I was still attempting to create a mental image of what I might see when I reached the patient.

"Did it really say eye?" I asked, already on my feet.

“That’s what I heard,” a deputy said as he shoved the door buzzer. “We’ve called for Code 3 Fire Department and ambulance response.”

As I scampered into the Women’s building, the deputies in Control who unlock doors, process visitors, and give directions to man-downs told me that the inmate was “Eliann, 28 years old, four months in. Schizophrenia, and has already been in jail several times in her short life. You know her.”

Another nurse, Alice, asked to accompany me to the “man down.” Alice is a 40-something single mom with 15 years of paramedic training followed by several years as an RN in the Trauma ICU at my beloved County Medical Center. She has residual PTSD resulting from her years as a paramedic and shares her diagnosis openly with her coworkers.

I jogged down the hall to the Women's building Medical office to collect a blood pressure cuff, adrenaline already pushing ahead of reason. Alice grabbed dressing supplies and dashed towards Eliann's cell.

When I reached Eliann, she was quietly and calmly sitting on her bunk, back straight, blood streaking down her cheek.

“Eliann,” I said softly, “can you hear me?”

She turned her head. Her left eye dangled, tethered by tissue.

Alice crouched. “Don’t move, sweetheart. I’m going to cover it”

The deputies were required to take many pictures of the injury and pictures of Eliann herself before we could dress the wound. So we waited a moment for the pictures to finish before Alice began cleaning the wound; the left eye was hanging down out of the eye socket. Alice applied a normal saline dampened 4x4 over the eye and socket and wrapped a Kerlix around her head to keep it in place.

Elian’s voice was flat, almost casual. “The scripture says, if your eye causes you to sin, pluck it out. Better to go to heaven with one eye than with two.”

My throat tightened. “You......you did this to yourself?”

"Like this." She lifted her right hand, demonstrating the motion.

Alice and I locked eyes. Neither of us spoke.

I looked at Eliann's hands; it was evident, from the appearance of her fingernails, that she had not been practicing good personal hygiene.

Boots thundered down the hall. Eliann became anxious as the Fire Department quickly arrived. The actual injury wasn't bloody, but the act itself of self-harm sent a wave of shock through the responding deputies, sergeants, lieutenants, nurses, mental health, Fire, and ambulance staff. While Alice and I attended to Eliann, the number of staff responding to the emergency totaled 18 people outside the cell. The rest of the dorm was "locked down" in their cells during the emergency.

The Fire Dept. asked the deputies what her charges were, so as to document a possible reason why she would do this.

"What are her charges?" one asked.

"County hold. Nothing violent," a deputy answered.

Another firefighter turned to me: "Medical history?"

"Schizophrenia. Medication compliant," I responded.

We provided the patient's medical history and mental health diagnosis for their documentation. She always took her meds every night – to treat decreased emotional expression, social withdrawal, and apathy.

Eliann sat quietly on her bunk as the deputies handcuffed her for transport to the ER. She was calm; her blood pressure was 112/72 and her pulse was 61. I'm sure my BP and pulse were through the roof during this experience; at least my heart felt like it would burst out of my chest.

Alice pressed gauze gently against Eliann's cheek. "Vitals are stable. She's calm. Let's keep her that way."

The gurney rattled down the hall, taking her away. The silence that followed pressed like a weight.

Later in the medical office, the staff circled, restless.

"Never seen anything like that," one deputy muttered, rubbing his temples.

Alice exhaled, "And I've seen plenty. But this..." She let the sentence die.

"You okay?" someone asked me.

"Yeah," I lied.

But when I sat down to chart, my hands shook so hard I could barely type. Still, the words went in: vitals, history, transport. The note became armor; if the facts lined up, maybe the memory would, too.

I filled out the paperwork to transmit to the ER. We had electronic medical records (EMR), but there was still paperwork involved when transporting to the ER. Medical history, allergies, current diagnoses, current medications, and a description of the emergency. A few years later, we upgraded to a much better EMR, but the ER staff couldn't access patients in custody, so we still continued working with a wad of paperwork.

The whole experience was shocking to all staff who responded. The dorm was so quiet you could hear a pin drop! I called my beloved Medical Center's ER to give Report to the Charge Nurse.

After Eliann was transported to the ER, Alice insisted we debrief. After so many years as a paramedic, Alice encouraged all nurses to share their feelings following traumatic experiences with inmates before the crews began to debrief between calls. The rest of the night was a blur; I kept trying to understand what Eliann had done. It was all I could think about.

The Mental Health staff joined the nurses during our dinner break to debrief as well. The therapist who responded knew Eliann and was surprised at her behavior. Once she understood what had happened, a decision was made to create a 5150 for Eliann after she was cleared by the ER because this was clearly an attempt to self-harm. The debriefing continued for several days; it was a comforting feeling to have coworkers there to talk about it and help make it less horrifying.

After her release from acute psych back to Oakwood, Eliann's vision was fine. She developed an orbital cellulitis, which was treated with antibiotics after the injury. She was also allowed to read the Bible. But the deputies needed to keep a closer eye on her.

Afterward, I felt hollowed out. I couldn't sleep. I returned to Mental Health again and again, desperate to unload the weight of what I'd seen. The trauma of managing her care left deep emotional scars on all of us, and I eventually needed support to cope. Some trauma doesn't fade—it burrows in.

I ended up seeing a psychiatrist after this trauma because it started interfering with my sleep. I explained to the psychiatrist what had happened. He was a little surprised; he admitted one of his patients had done the same thing, but he wasn't there at the time. He concluded that this event gave me a bit of PTSD and ordered a few benzos for sleep. Eventually, a few months later, I began sleeping without interruptions.

I relayed this incident to my mental health friend, Jelly, who wasn't at work the day it happened. She was somewhat upset hearing about the details of Eliann's actions.

We dealt with our stress the best way we knew how...we sent funny things to each other. Once again, we exchanged silly stockings. We had worked our way through the maze of animal icons, complete with pictures of kittens, to holiday themes like Santa Claus and the Easter Bunny, and had now transitioned to "statement socks." My first pair of statement socks simply said, "WTF?" Whenever I wore these socks to work, I snickered and giggled, knowing the three letters hidden under my scrubs had my back, so to speak.

Jelly and I also made videos wearing our "I'm a f*cking delicate flower" socks; and the videos were sophisticated, as well. Jelly sent me a video from her exercise class showing the shock and dismay from her classmates! So I took my "delicate flower" socks on the road; my video showed them stuck out the window while riding as a passenger down the freeway (no, not in the back seat of a self-driving vehicle!). We had lots of laughs and felt our stress melt away.

> ***Laughter is the best medicine.***
> ***But if you're laughing for no reason,***
> ***you may need medicine.***
> *-Dr. Oz*

Divya

A petite, soft-spoken East Indian woman looked almost breakable standing alone in the crowded dorm, trying to navigate jail culture amid fear and unfamiliar customs. She struggled with cultural dietary restrictions and was losing weight quickly. In a whisper, she told me other inmates had taken food as payment for helping her fill out commissary forms. When we helped her move to safer housing and arranged proper support, she looked at me with a raw gratitude that tightened my throat. Sometimes the bravest thing someone can do in jail is ask for help.

I met an East Indian patient named Divya at pill call one evening in the minimum dorm.

I would come to find out what big challenges this tiny woman had had since her arrest.

Divya declined her meds and complained about her diet. She reported her inability to eat the jail food and had difficulty swallowing. She said it had been three weeks since she was arrested and brought to Oakwood. I had her come out for assessments after pill call so I could speak to her at length about her problems with her diet. She was East Indian, in her 30s, under 5 feet tall, thin, and had difficulty making contact with her parents, which was stressing her out.

I purposely waited until I had completed my other assessments to meet with Divya because I anticipated a longer interaction with her. She repeatedly complained about needing her Indian medicine for her chronic neck pain. She had been seen in the clinic, and the MD had ordered an NSAID, as needed, for pain. Nonsteroidal anti-inflammatory drugs (NSAIDs) are a group of medicines that relieve pain and fever and reduce inflammation. NSAIDs include aspirin and several generic ibuprofen products, including brand names Advil, Motrin, and Nuprin.

She had met with the chaplain, who could authorize a vegetarian diet for religious reasons. She complained that potatoes, pasta, and bread were not part of her regular diet. All she could eat were the carrots. So the chaplain authorized the special vegetarian diet.

At her appointment with Medical, she requested a low-salt, low-fat diet so she could get rice. But the MD refused her request because she didn't have a history of hypertension or high cholesterol. The MD also informed her that Indian medicine was not used at Oakwood. I was quite concerned when we weighed her that she had lost another pound in the past three days. Her booking weight had been 120 pounds. Her current weight was 105 pounds. With her tiny, short, and thin stature, her jail-issue extra-small (XS) clothes were dangerously loose and had to be rolled up and tucked in to mitigate the tripping hazard.

I formulated a plan to get the dietitian to meet with Divya about her dietary needs. To get my request authorized, I told the Nurse Manager the unusual situation Divya was experiencing.

As I described my plan to Divya, a look of fear and panic developed in her eyes. The deputy standing by during assessments moved closer as she explained what had happened to her a few days prior. For more privacy, the deputy, Divya, and I moved to the inner treatment room so none of the trustees passing by in the hall could listen to our conversation.

Divya had been moved from one dorm to another earlier that day. She reported that a couple of the seasoned, older inmates had offered to "help her" fill out her commissary form. When her commissary was delivered, these women took it all for "payment."

They then threw her bedding on the floor and threw towels at her. Divya said that they called her an "engineer bitch." She told us how she tried to teach these ladies that they couldn't treat people like that, and also tried to convince them to change their foul language.

It was obvious Divya didn't understand how things worked in jail. The deputies immediately changed her housing for her safety.

After speaking with her for 30 minutes, the deputy and I informed Divya we needed to come up with a plan. I suggested referring her to one of our MH therapists who might be able to help with her adjustment challenges. The deputy planned to move her to a more readily observable bunk for her safety. I let my manager know this patient had not been eating much for three weeks, but it wasn't a hunger strike; it was a cultural dietary issue.

During the entire 30 minutes, Divya referred to the deputy as "ma'am." She was so grateful for the time we took with her to listen and come up with a plan, that she knelt down and touched the toe of the deputy's boot to give her thanks as though she was bowing to a Queen.

In my 15 years as a nurse at Oakwood Medical, this was my first and only experience with an East Indian female (very rare) at the Oakwood jail, and the challenges that their culture, dietary preferences, and social differences present in the jail setting.

She was so completely different from any other patient I had at Oakwood. After these events, she would be watched more closely by Medical for her dietary issues and by the deputies for safety reasons. I never saw her again.

Sometimes the bravest thing someone can do in jail is to simply ask for help. Helping her find safer housing and proper support reaffirmed how small interventions can change someone's entire experience.

> ***You can't change how people treat you***
> ***or what they say about you.***
> ***All you can do is change***
> ***how you react to it.***
>
> *- Mahatma Gandhi*

Ennis

Ennis arrived in severe withdrawal, his suffering filling the dorm. For nearly five hours, he screamed for help, shaking as his mind unraveled. Deputies paced, nurses exchanged weary glances, and I felt the strain of trying to steady someone splintering apart. When he finally stabilized, it felt like a storm passing — leaving wreckage behind. It was one of the hardest detox cases I ever handled, and a stark reminder of how deeply withdrawal can shake a unit.

It was October 30, the night before Halloween, my favorite holiday. On this cold, dreary night, Oakwood was not joyful.

Ennis was just 24 when he arrived at Oakwood Medical, having been transferred from Lockdown. You could tell right away that he was struggling; he was in the middle of a tough detox from Xanax, heroin, and alcohol, and it showed. His eyes were wide, and he looked exhausted. He cried out repeatedly for hours, "Please, help me!" His desperate pleas echoed through the building, making it hard for anyone to find what little peace could exist in the place. It was heartbreaking and disrupted the already tense atmosphere, affecting everyone around him.

He had been started on symptom management medication for alcohol withdrawal, stomach upset, diarrhea, generalized pain, and sleep. Ennis was placed in a private room near the Medical Deputy by the Charge Nurse. He was shackled to a gurney and given a blanket, some ice water, and soda crackers. But Ennis continued to yell. He began at 6 p.m. and continued to scream, "Please, help me!," despite repeated attempts to calm him down and reminders that he had received all the medication he could get for now.

One of the nurses called the on-call MD and got a telephone order to start an IV for hydration. The IV was started. Some nurses saw him stick his finger down his throat to induce vomiting.

A seasoned deputy who started his shift at 6 p.m. voiced safety concerns. A disruptive patient in Medical can distract the deputy and divert his attention from all patients coming to Medical for blood pressure checks, wound care, neuro checks after head injuries, etc. We had counted as many as 60 invitations sent to inmates to report to Medical at the same time – 7 p.m.

After an hour of Ennis constantly yelling out, "Please, help me!," I approached him and asked him to stop yelling so I could talk to him. I was Charge Nurse that night, and answering phone calls was almost impossible with the continuous yelling in the background. I shared with him the new program recently initiated to help heroin addicts with their withdrawal. He listened quietly as I explained how individual patients would be evaluated for withdrawal symptoms. These symptoms are scored on the COWS (Clinical Opiate Withdrawal Scale).

The protocol mandates housing in the Infirmary downtown and five days of Suboxone. Ennis perked up when he heard this! He had been given Suboxone to taper off heroin in a previous situation. "I had Suboxone before, and I want it now!" he yelled. I tried calmly to explain to him that at 7 p.m. there were no MDs on site to initiate the Suboxone protocol.

He adamantly refused to wait, and the non-stop yelling resumed. In my 15 years at Oakwood Medical, I had never had this level of disruption from a patient detoxing from multiple medications. The on-call MD, one of the MDs authorized to initiate Suboxone for patients, was paged for other issues. She could hear him over the phone in the background and requested the nurses draw labs to rule out abdominal issues that may interfere with starting the protocol on him. The on-call MD agreed that if he was exceedingly difficult, we should send him to the ER in the back of a patrol car.

The nurses approached Ennis to draw labs as he continued to yell. The deputy was concerned for the nurses' safety. I asked the nurses, "Do you feel safe drawing his blood?" They each indicated, "I don't feel comfortable in this situation."

Oakwood Control was called to request a patrol car to transport a patient in Medical who needed labs drawn, but was too disruptive for the nurses, and needed to go to the ER, where trained staff members could help get the labs drawn safely. Oakwood Control is in charge of opening gates, notifying the Fire Department of Code 3 emergencies, keeping track of inmates at the hospital, and keeping track of the deputies with them. Requesting a patrol car was not an emergency. It might be two hours before a deputy would be available for this run to the ER.

We were approaching two straight hours of yelling. Ennis didn't like it when told his behavior would delay the process. A half-hour later, he agreed to let the nurses draw his blood. "We need to expedite the process," he insisted. It was surprising to hear this language used by Ennis, who looked like a young adult but acted like a child.

The blood was drawn, but Ennis still didn't want to wait. He exclaimed, "I'm going to have a psychotic breakdown!" For hours on end, his haunting cries filled the building, each plea laced with desperation and anguish.

A Mental Health referral was hand-carried to the office. Three staff members were standing and chatting. I explained the situation, and they laughed at me. I turned around to leave, planning to send a sharply worded email about staff response to my request to the Medical and the MH managers. Then one turned to me and said, "I'll take the referral." After reading about the patient's booking history, the Mental Health staff member walked down the hall to notify me that his name was added to "the list." He gently explained they couldn't do anything while the inmate was in the process of detoxing. As he stood there, Ennis continued yelling. I was grateful when the staff offered to speak with Ennis.

Around 10 p.m. – the cutoff time to contact the on-call MD – the on-call MD called and could hear Ennis continue to yell (now four hours later). The MD agreed to have him transferred to the Infirmary in anticipation of starting the Suboxone taper in the morning. All of his stat labs measured within normal limits, which ruled out pancreatitis. The cries had lasted for a total of 4.5 hours. I felt so sad to think Ennis had behaved like this. Something was wrong. Even after Ennis was transferred to the Infirmary, the sound of his yelling continued to ring in my ears.

It was one of the most difficult detox cases I ever handled, and showed how deeply withdrawal can shake a unit. All of the heroin addicts I had met previous to him were quiet, gentle individuals who "kicked" alone and quietly, suffering without all the noise. I genuinely hope Ennis can get the help he needs in his life. As the seasoned deputy in Medical said, "In my 25 years here at Oakwood, this is the worst night shift I've ever had."

> ***If you have to choose between being kind***
> ***and being right,***
> ***choose being kind, and you will always be right.***
> *- HealthyPlace.com*

Mama Fay

One homeless elder was a force — part street angel, part prophet, part weary survivor. She told vivid stories of protecting children, organizing clothing drives, and standing up for those no one else saw. But woven through them were threads of paranoia and exhaustion that broke my heart. She carried trauma and tenderness like twin weights. Listening to her reminded me how easily elders slip through society's cracks — protecting others while desperately needing protection themselves.

Mama Fay had been arrested and jailed. She was housed in a maximum-security single cell and did not interact with other inmates. Betty, part of the Mental Health staff, was interviewing Mama to assess her ability to deal with and attempt to overcome her problems.

Betty slid into the chair across from Mama Fay's narrow cot. Clipboard balanced on her knee, she clicked her pen and asked gently, "How are you coping, Fay?"

Mama Fay sat forward, her wiry hands resting on her knees. "The air in here—it's bad. No fresh air, no sunlight. I'm locked up in this tiny cell. They don't even open that little hatch where they shove the food through." Her voice rose, bouncing off the cement walls. "I only get out every other day, one hour. In that short time, I gotta shower, clean, and get my water. I wash out my own clothes. No time to even step out onto that little cement square they call a sun deck."

She rubbed her eyes, red-rimmed and tired. "They took away my eyedrops. Don't know why. I'll just make do. My eyes burn. My stomach's bleeding, I'm throwing up blood. Got fleas. Lice." She suddenly stood and smacked the wall, crushing a spider with her palm.

"And these damn things crawling around! Probably what's been biting us." She glared. "Don't you dare write that down."

Betty held her pen still. "Why do you think you've been here so long?"

"Six months," Mama Fay barked. "For what? I don't drink, I'm no prostitute. I'm celibate—my body is sacred. They said I spit on an officer. Why would I spit? My saliva belongs in me. And besides, I don't even know how to spit! He lied." Her jaw clenched. "I can't stand liars. There's a ton of liars in here. Some of these COs are mean and crooked. Some are nice. but too many lie."

Her tone softened for a moment. "Out on the streets, the cops come to me. They say, 'Mama Fay, help us find the guy who did this – or that. Help us track that one.' And I do. We know the streets, the people. We help. I always said: Do the crime, do the time. I think it's better for some person or kid who is going bad or doing wrong things to go to jail and put a stop to it. I believe in just punishment and doing your time."

"But me? I didn't do no crime. They're after me 'cause I speak for the houseless."

She lifted her chin proudly. "Not 'homeless.' You can have a home anywhere. The Earth is our home. They're houseless. A lot of the problem started when Reagan closed those mental institutions and left folks with nowhere to go. They should be taken care of in hospitals."

"I did not seek out this position. I never asked to be their spokesperson, but the newspaper came, took my picture." I told 'em, 'Don't focus on me, focus on them, focus on her out there. That's your story – not me.'"

"But I'll admit, they got a good picture of me." She smiled faintly. "We're trying to open a center, run by us street people. I got over 700 signatures to support us."

Her eyes sharpened. "I'm safe on the streets. People look after me, and I look after them. Once, two young girls came running. 'Mama

Fay, that man's trying to pimp us!' I stood in front of him. Told him, 'They're my daughters. You get out of here now.' He hit me in the face. First and only time I've been hurt. I counsel the young ones. I steer them away from the junk, away from the crime. I help them straighten out their lives. I do not support drug use. I do not support criminal activity."

She leaned back, remembering. "Last Christmas, people dropped off piles of blankets, clothes, and sleeping bags. I guarded it all night. Frostbitten fingers. Couldn't leave it. Handed things out fair and square. Anyone could have anything they wanted, and often turned in what they had so someone else could use it. Folks thought I was crazy. Maybe I was, but I couldn't leave that stuff. Nobody went without."

Betty scribbled notes. "Tell me about your family, Fay."

"I had a good home once. My grandmother taught me Native ways – yes, I'm Native American, Irish, and Black. I honor my family and the generations before me. I was taught the sacred ways. I was trained in ballet. I still dance in the park. My body remembers. Dancing is the way I express myself. I tell a story through form and movement.

"I grew up in New York State, out on the island with many different people: Italian, Puerto Rican, Black, Hispanic, Korean, all kinds. But I say the Asians should go back to where they came from. The guy who arrested me was Asian."

Her face darkened suddenly. "But this land is ours, the tribes here. Others should stay where they belong. I know we are all different tribes and in the end we'll all be together as one people, but for now the North American Continent is MY land and they should go back to where they came from."

She muttered curses, half to herself, half to God. "He knows what's in my mouth before I speak it. If I curse, it's to get people's attention. That's between me and Him. Right now, I'm mad at God. Why am I here? I'm so sick of this and tired and can't stand it. My people on the street think I deserted them. They don't know I'm trapped in here."

A sharp knock cut through the room. A deputy leaned in. "There's a 415 – an altercation. Mama Fay needs to lock down."

As Betty stood, promising to return, Mama Fay lunged at the door. Her foot slammed against the steel, screaming, "Go back to your own country, you 'friggin g***'!" The rest blurred into a howl of rage as the door clanged shut.

Betty's final note would read:

Introduction to Precious Grace, Queen of the downtown homeless. Unofficial spokesperson for the houseless, the disenfranchised, and official momma figure and dispenser of wisdom to street people who are drug addicts, or girls who would even think of selling their bodies. Not on HER watch.

> ***Choose your words wisely.***
> ***Time and patience are your tickets to a healthy and successful transaction.***
> ***Once words are said, they can only be forgiven, not forgotten.***
>
> *- Arthur Rubinstein*

Adventures in Lockdown

The fistfight erupted so fast I barely had time to think. One moment, I was waiting for pill call to start; the next, I was sprinting into a locked restroom, adrenaline surging as fists flew behind me. Later, a seasoned deputy admitted his fear that new nurses could be manipulated or blindsided in these high-risk units. His honesty pushed me to report the systemic gaps putting us all at risk. In jail, safety wasn't guaranteed — it had to be fought for.

Every shift at Oakwood is unique. No matter your role, you must be ready for anything.

The deputies often ask us to check patients with medical complaints they are concerned about. We check patients with mental health issues and do a full assessment to rule out medical issues before calling MH. Sometimes, there are disagreements between Medical and MH regarding detox issues. If alcohol or opiates are involved, the inmates generally stay under Medical care. Patients may complain of detox symptoms from a change in a mental health medication (usually lowering a dose). Medical will continue to monitor those patients for safety.

A female inmate complained about the food and stopped eating. She insisted there was something in her food that shouldn't be there. MH assessed that the patient was not suicidal and cleared her, meaning she was safe to remain in the unit. But she still wasn't eating. The deputies were alerted to watch her eat; she would sometimes flush her food down the toilet to make it look like she had eaten her meal. This went on for several weeks.

One of our brightest nurses took a good look at the patient one night and had a bad feeling. She sought out an esteemed mental health therapist and explained the patient's history. The therapist made arrangements to transfer the patient to the Acute Psych Unit downtown so the staff could keep a closer eye on her. After being there a couple of days, the patient became unresponsive and stopped breathing. Staff performed CPR and sent the patient to the ER. She was put on a ventilator, IVs, and dialysis. She eventually recovered from her malnutrition and dehydration.

***

I was assigned to a lockdown building. Each building has four different dorms. The nurses on the 3-11 shift go out to their assignments before the inmates eat dinner to check the diabetics' blood sugars and give medications due for that time.

This particular evening, I was returning to the male lockdown unit at 7 p.m. to start passing evening medication. This building had many patients who had been in jail for a long time, fighting their cases. I approached the Control deputy of the building, who is aware of issues in the dorms (shakedowns, interviews, etc). Control dictated the order of the dorms for pill call.

After a couple of hours, I finally was ready to start the fourth and final dorm of the building to complete pill call. I pushed my medication cart and blood pressure machine into the dorm for those patients who needed to have their vital signs checked during pill call.

The deputy had everyone locked down. Now, pill call is done according to groups. He unlocked specific cells by pushing buttons on a control panel on the wall behind his desk. In each dorm, the DOC Classification Department determines whether inmates are safe to be housed in the same dorm, but there are still inmates who are "keep aways" within that same dorm. These factors are all taken into consideration during pill call. The deputy looks at the control panel to determine whether certain cells are locked before unlocking the next set of cells to proceed with pill call. As the deputy is unlocking the cell doors for pill call, his back is momentarily turned away from the dorm.

I had my medication cart safely situated next to the deputy's desk. I waited for the deputy to unlock the cells to begin pill call. His back was turned away from the dorm. I was at the medication cart, facing out toward the dorm.

I noticed two inmates I assumed were trustees starting to actually punch each other in the dorm. I had never been this close to a fight and was surprised it was so quiet. It took me a moment to realize it was an altercation. I called out, "Deputy, 415, 415!" 415 is the code the DOC uses to describe a disruptive behavior, loud argument, or fight. The deputy turned to see the inmates and called for help on the radio. He then approached the inmates cautiously as he waited for backup. I ran into the bathroom located directly behind the deputy's desk and locked the door. This is a safety technique the nurses are taught in case of an emergency in the dorms. I heard the commotion as more deputies ran into the dorm from all over Oakwood. The Sergeant called my name a few minutes later, saying it was safe for me to come out of the restroom.

After debriefing the Sergeant about the incident, I was asked to medically clear the two inmates involved in the altercation. They were handcuffed and seated in separate cells. Pill call was delayed as inmates were interviewed about the altercation. The dorm deputy was interviewed for his statement, and all of the other inmates in the dorm were "locked down" (locked in their cells). Pill call eventually resumed, but not with the usual line of inmates to receive medications. To be safe, the deputy released just one inmate at a time. When one inmate closed his cell door, the next inmate was let out.

I had been working at Oakwood Medical for 13 years when this happened. I had been a first responder to altercations in dorms I'd been assigned to many times. The difference this time was that the altercation had begun right in front of me! This occurrence brings to mind all of the emails, announcements, and newspaper articles regarding the increased number of inmates at Oakwood because of AB109, which directed that those released from prison on parole be returned back to the local jails where they were sent after being arrested. We were told these inmates were more sophisticated and dangerous after spending time in prison. The risk of threatening situations faced by nurses certainly keeps our adrenaline pumping.

***

A few months later, I was assigned to a different male inmate lockdown building. A deputy approached me. He had more than 20 years of experience between Oakwood and the downtown jail, where the maximum-security male inmates are housed. He had been involved in deputy training for most of his career. Ask any deputy at Oakwood; they will all agree this deputy had their back!

He approached me because he knew I'd been working at Oakwood Medical for a while. He brought up a recent incident where the nurse had their iPhone stolen off the medication cart. I agreed with him that it was not only against the rules to have your phone with you during pill call, but that it was a security issue that an inmate or inmates had gotten hold of this item. (Update: The stolen iPhone was returned the same day.)

The deputy said, "I have tremendous concerns over nurses' safety here in the jail. I am concerned the new nurses aren't taught appropriate safety techniques when working with this population. Some nurses are even shopping for personal items for inmates!" I was stunned; I had no idea nurses were shopping for inmates.

After I finished my shift, I sent an email to our nursing supervisor and nurse manager detailing the deputy's concerns. As the unofficial safety monitor for Oakwood Medical, I also notified our union reps. Working in a jail setting is dangerous. Prisoners can be manipulative and threatening.

The Oakwood Safety Deputy encourages new hires to read "Downing of a Duck." The prison jargon "duck" refers to an institution employee who can be manipulated or easily fooled. Inmates have a process they use to manipulate staff to get them to do what they want. This reading material is a first-hand narrative from a prisoner skilled in the art of "turning" his jailers so they'd work for him, bringing in drugs, money, booze, and contraband.

The Safety Deputy counters this by teaching staff to identify games criminals play. "We want to prevent staff from over-identifying with the inmates." One way of doing so is to report everything. "I'd rather have staff over-report," he advocates. "If it quacks, it's probably a duck."

> ***Yesterday's the past,***
> ***tomorrow's the future,***
> ***but today is a gift.***
> ***That's why it's called the present.***
> *- Bill Keane*

Leigh

Leigh drifted in and out of jail like a ghost — fragile, unhoused, schizophrenic, and living with Type 1 diabetes in a body that seemed tired of trying. After stabilization, she could be sweet and chatty, sharing stories with soft eyes. Other times, she arrived dehydrated, confused, and refusing care as her blood sugars soared. Each time she left custody, I wondered whether the world outside would swallow her whole.

An inmate/patient I will never forget is Leigh, a 20-something young lady with curly blonde hair who was an intermittent visitor to the ladies' Special Management dorm. Leigh not only had a "life sentence" of Type 1 diabetes, but she also carried a diagnosis of schizophrenia. Oh, there was one more significant, unpredictable, and horrifying item on her plate: she was homeless!

I was awed by her ability to survive these several unforgiving challenges in her life. For those of you who aren't familiar with the homeless population, a young, healthy woman who is homeless faces extraordinary danger daily because of the darkness that lives in that community. I always thought she should be equipped with large orange cones stationed at her feet, surrounding her to provide an extra layer of protection.

Whenever Leigh would arrive in the dorm from the streets, she was off all of her meds. Her blood sugars were in the four hundreds, and her unmedicated mental health issues made communication with her impossible. All female inmates must have a negative pregnancy test before starting on medications. But Leigh violently refused blood sugar testing, the urine specimen for a pregnancy test, the urine test for ketones, and any interaction in general when she first arrived at Oakwood after she was booked.

High levels of ketones in the urine indicate diabetic ketoacidosis, which, untreated, can lead to death. Testing for ketones is part of the diabetic protocol. We tried to get the Mental Health (MH) staff to transfer her to the Acute Psych Unit because she refused to participate in the diabetic protocol, but it frequently fell on deaf ears. MH staff referred inmates to the Psych Unit for being a danger to themselves or a danger to others, not for medical issues. The nurses had to involve MDs for her to be transferred to the Psychiatric Unit for better control of her medical and mental health issues.

After several days on the unit, Leigh would return to the Special Management dorm feeling like herself again – friendly and compliant with her diabetic regimen and taking her MH medication. It was always nice to see her somewhat groomed and speaking in complete sentences again.

"Hi, nurse," she said. "How are you?"

I replied, "I'm happy to see you again, Leigh." She had a happy twinkle in her eyes, an indicator that she was feeling better on her meds.

The last few times Leigh was booked, she had open sores, usually on her legs. A Type 1 diabetic with poorly controlled blood sugar has great difficulty healing wounds. After Leigh did her time at the Psychiatric facility, she returned to Oakwood. We asked her about the nature of the wounds, which weren't dressed because of her combativeness until she was back on her medications. She could never remember how she developed the lesions. The look on her face was so innocent. I left work still thinking about how vulnerable she was in the homeless community. She insisted that being homeless was okay. She didn't have any family who could provide housing for her. Leigh was a survivor.

A couple of years passed, and Leigh no longer showed up at Oakwood. I worried that her luck had run out. Every time I saw an article in the newspaper about a woman found dead near downtown, I feared it was Leigh.

This young lady made a big impression on me. She had many challenges in her life, yet she wasn't bitter or angry. Once she was back on her medications, she just dealt with what life had handed her with grace.

I hope Leigh is living life with all the good things she deserves.

> ***Don't be pushed around by the fears***
> ***in your mind.***
> ***Be led by the dreams in your heart.***
> *- Roy T. Bennett*

Gentle Giant aka The Enforcer

He towered over everyone. Yet when he spoke to me, it was with a quiet respect that softened the room. His blood pressure ran dangerously high, but he refused medication, leaving us monitoring him for hours. Beneath his size and his record was a boy shaped by a world that had offered few safe choices.

Danny made quite an impression on me the first time we met. He stood 6'5" and weighed 300 lb.; a mountain of muscle and menace. This young man, in his thirties, interacted with the nurses at a level of respect we didn't usually experience at Oakwood. The nurses needed to see him often due to a new diagnosis of hypertension. He refused to take his prescription because he believed the medicine caused brown spots on his legs.

We took his blood pressure. It measured 170/100. He was completely asymptomatic. Our protocol for patients with a blood pressure greater than 140/90 is to have them wait in the Medical Lobby with a plastic water pitcher, where they sip for 30-45 minutes. Once the patient has consumed the water, the nurses recheck their blood pressure in 15-minute increments. The patient can be medically "cleared" to return to his barracks after his blood pressure registers less than 140/90. The time it took to clear him varied. If we checked him after commissary, it took up to two hours to clear him because most of the food contained large quantities of salt.

Danny frequently tried to hide the empty water pitcher in his pants to take it back to the barracks, a prized possession for any lucky new owner. It could be traded for cigarettes or commissary. But the deputies always caught him and forced him to give it up. This was repeated several times. He got all the lectures about high blood pressure and stroke. He told the nurses that his father told him not to "take the white man's medicine." Danny's heritage included African American, Latino, and Asian.

Nurse Dana had known Danny all his life. According to Dana, both his parents were drug addicts, and he was drawn into the family business. His aunt helped take care of him as a child. As he grew up, he alienated her with his continued drug use. Despite the life he'd been dealt, he knew to be respectful of the nurses.

I made an appointment for Danny to see one of the Oakwood MDs in an upcoming clinic to discuss his medical issues. I usually tell patients when I am scheduling an appointment for them. If they are being sent an invitation to go to Medical for an MD appointment and don't know why, they are more likely to refuse.

On the day of his appointment, I found out during the change of shift Report that he had complained of chest pain and been sent Code 3 to the ER. He had been sent to the ER for hypertension before this episode; the trip was like a short reprieve from jail. A brief trip. He knew how the system worked. Before I learned the details, I thought he might have even called his family or girlfriend for a quick reunion in the ER.

But Danny was not seen at my beloved Medical Center. The ambulance was diverted to a different hospital because our ER had too many patients. So I couldn't look up the details of his visit because the notes weren't on our computer. I understood that he was seen and cleared. His blood pressure had stabilized. He was now on his way back to Oakwood. Working at the front desk at Medical that evening, I was looking forward to seeing the ER notes. The deputy carried a paper copy of the visit report.

An hour passed, and he wasn't back. I opened his chart.

Custody had moved him to the Main Jail downtown. I called the Booking nurse, who assesses the new bookings and medically clears patients returning from the hospital.

The Booking nurse said something about an altercation!

I asked the deputies in Medical what happened. They reported that Danny was part of a group of large inmates who had roughed up another inmate the night before. The injured inmate came to Medical, but he fabricated the cause of his injuries. He knew if he gave up the names of the guys who beat him up, the next beating would be worse.

The deputies checked the cameras in the barracks. Danny was one of three inmates who beat up the injured inmate. Custody rolled him up to the Main Jail to face new charges. Our gentle giant in Oakwood Medical was a bad guy.

I saw Dana later that night and told her what had happened to him. Dana matter-of-factly replied, "He's The Enforcer. He's always been the big guy who beats people up."

The Enforcer. My heart is broken for this gentle giant who seemed so polite and respectful in Medical. He never revealed the "Enforcer" side to the nurses.

I still remember the last time I saw the Gentle Giant.

He had quietly said to me, "Thank you for everything."

> ***Forget what hurt you.***
> ***But never forget what it taught you.***
> *- lovethispic.com*

The Good, the Bad, and the Ugly

I arrived that day already depleted, overwhelmed by the workload, only to be dismissed by a supervisor who saw me as "not full-time" and therefore less deserving of grace. The sting lingered — until a traumatic patient event unraveled me completely. It was Ana, another nurse, who held space for my tears and anger. In jail, management support was inconsistent, but the solidarity among nurses saved me again and again.

I had just arrived at work for the 3-11:30 PM shift and was getting ready to go to the ladies' minimum/medium security building to check the diabetics before dinner.

Working with these ladies could be challenging, and had been for the last few days. We usually had the same assignment for two weeks. Besides the work I had been assigned for each evening, I found myself doing additional work (assessing patient medical issues) that should have been done before I arrived, and things turned ugly. (Though that wasn't the "ugly" part of this particular day...)

I complained to my supervisor that the assignment was unusually heavy (a rarity for me). She turned to me and said, "Why are you complaining?...You don't even work full-time."

It was true. I worked seven days every two weeks. Before working at Oakwood, I had worked for 20 years in home care & hospice. We had the most supportive bosses at that time. That was my real problem. I had recently worked in a wonderful, supportive environment, and I expected it to happen again!

I was headed out to the ladies' building for diabetic call when the Charge Nurse asked me the question that started the event that made me question my nursing experience.

An 18-year-old lady had recently been booked. She had told the Booking nurse she needed to have her medication verified at Stanford. She identified as a transgender individual and was receiving hormone injections. The Booking nurse documented in her medical record that she didn't have a vagina. I was asked to interview the inmate to determine their gender so they could be properly housed.

I imagined speaking to the patient as I walked to the building. What would I say to maintain respect for the patient while obtaining the information I needed? I had never experienced an interaction like this with any of the patients I had met in my years as a nurse. I had studied Anatomy and Physiology in school, but never had to ask a patient to show me their lady/man parts to confirm their gender.

I was directed to a holding cell. I opened the heavy metal door and found a tiny African American young lady sitting quietly on the bench. I took a deep breath and informed her in the gentlest voice I had to verify the information she had given to the Booking nurse.

Ms. Tucker emphatically stated, "I told them I *do* have a vagina!" I sheepishly apologized for the inconvenience. I quietly informed the deputies on the unit that she confirmed that she had a vagina.

Then I left the unit and headed to the Medical office to begin diabetic call. Before that, I quickly called the Women's Sergeant to inform her the patient reported she had a vagina. The sergeant asked if I had visually determined the gender of the patient by performing an examination. I replied, "No. I have never done that while working at Oakwood Medical." I also called my less-than-supportive supervisor to inform her that the patient told me she had a vagina.

My supervisor said she would call the sergeant. I didn't know it yet, but the next phone call would start the "bad" part of my shift. My supervisor called back to say the sergeant wanted a visual examination of the inmate to determine their gender. Don't get me wrong, I've been "down there" many times to insert urinary catheters. But this was the first time I had to report the sex of a patient to a sergeant.

Now things were turning "ugly" for me. Again, I had *never* had to perform a visual examination of an inmate to determine sex. The supervisor was sending another nurse (Ana) to be a chaperone. Ana proved to be the voice of reason for me. I had to run through the "performance" of the examination before we called Ms. Tucker to our medical office. I felt like I was having an out-of-body experience.

I needed coaxing to determine how to ask Ms. Tucker to show me her female anatomy. My mouth was dry, and I was a little short of breath – adrenaline to the rescue. Ms. Tucker came into Medical. I asked the patient the prearranged questions to arrive at the inevitable stirrup position. Ms. Tucker wasn't as visibly upset as I'd anticipated. She reported that she was used to this type of exam. She got up on the exam table, covered her pelvis with the paper drape, leaned back, and assumed the position. (The door to Medical only had a privacy screen; no closed doors allowed.)Ana and I "determined" her gender. She got off the table, pulled up her pants, and quietly left the room. I called the sergeant to report a visual examination by Ana, and I confirmed that Ms. Tucker was female.

I then had to face the computer and document this unusual situation. Ana helped me put the words together to document her female gender. I came back to Oakwood Medical after diabetic call. I asked Della, my coworker, who had 25 years of experience at Oakwood, for help. In all her years at Oakwood Medical, Della also had *never* had to determine the gender of an inmate!

The "good" part of this whole fiasco was the support I got from Ana when I really needed it.

We spent time comparing stories of working in difficult situations with the inmates. I am actually glad it was my job to carry out this delicate interaction; being in jail for the first time must be scary enough! I know Ana and I were the most compassionate nurses available to help this young lady through this examination. The following week, the 3-11 p.m. shift would lose Ana to the day shift.

But I'm thankful that the Universe kept her on my shift long enough to help me through the good, the bad, and the ugly of it all.

Being challenged in life is inevitable.
Being defeated is optional.

- Roger Crawford

A Precious Commodity Behind Bars

Ice — just frozen water — became a quiet luxury behind bars. It soothed swollen joints, dulled tooth pain, and helped pregnant women rest. The filtered water tasted better than anything else available. When I had extra, I'd slip ice to favorite patients and watch their faces soften with relief. In a place stripped of comfort, even the smallest kindness can echo loudly.

Transitioning from diverse nursing backgrounds in hospitals, homecare, hospice, and after-hours advice to a correctional healthcare setting presented unique challenges. My professional experience had equipped me with specific protocols for managing patient care scenarios: identifying fever in post-operative patients, recognizing early wound infections, or addressing pain management and nausea in hospice settings. However, these decades of medical expertise only partially prepared me for the intricacies of nursing in a correctional facility like Oakwood.

The learning curve was significant. I needed to develop specialized skills in interacting with patients presenting psychiatric diagnoses and understanding their complex medication regimens. A critical component of my new role involved mastering the Standardized Procedures (SP) developed by MDs, which covered protocols for over-the-counter medications treating common conditions like upper respiratory infections, constipation, and allergies.

One frequently utilized Standardized Procedure focused on Muscle Soreness/Sprain management. Under specific guidelines, patients could receive Tylenol or NSAIDs for several days. When injury-related swelling was present and acute fractures were ruled out, patients were authorized to receive ice packs, applied three times daily for three consecutive days. Notably, the ice was produced from a filtered water machine, which tasted better than the water from the drinking fountains in the dorm.

I collected a few bags of ice before I left for pill call at night. Most nights, a patient was scheduled to receive a bag for a recent injury. Pregnant women received a bag of ice chips to prevent dehydration. If altercations occurred before or during pill call, an extra bag of ice could be immediately applied to the injury. When pill call was completed, patients would ask if there was any leftover ice. I have to admit I had my favorite patients who would be the first to receive the leftover ice; if they weren't interested and no one else showed an interest in the ice, I would leave it in the unit's freezer. There was usually a refrigerator in the buildings for the deputy's meals. Having ice in the freezer in the building furthest away from Medical was a time-saver for the nurses who needed ice during pill call.

Patients frequently put the unused ice in their drinks. The filtered water was actually delicious compared to the tap water in some of the older units. If there was leftover ice after commissary, it was added to the group's drinks and savored by all who tasted it. It didn't happen often, so inmates who got any leftover ice knew it was a special treat.

This detail illuminated the special nature of correctional healthcare – where seemingly mundane elements like ice distribution could provide small comforts; where each interaction represents an opportunity to recognize the human elements inherent in healthcare delivery to provide compassionate, standardized care amid the challenges of a jail setting.

> ***You only live once, but if you do it right, once is enough.***
>
> -Mae West

Somebody Came into my Cell!

He said someone had entered his cell and inserted something into his rectum while he slept. My mind tightened between suspicion and compassion. His paranoia complicated the story, but I couldn't dismiss him. Protocol required a PREA report, a doctor's consult, and an ER evaluation. He never returned for follow-up, and the loose ends lingered. In jail, truth is often a puzzle with missing pieces.

I was asked to meet with Charles, a 32-year-old gentleman who had complained in court earlier that day that he had a rectal abscess that needed attention. Occasionally, inmates will mention medical issues in court after requests for medical care fall on deaf ears. Then it becomes a "court order for medical care." After the patient receives care, a document defining the care given is faxed to the courts so the judge knows the court order was acknowledged and completed.

I introduced myself to Charles and explained that I was following up on what he'd told the judge. He sat in the chair in the medical office, nervously shifting back and forth in the seat. The deputy stood at the door for my safety. Charles took a deep breath and said, "Someone shoved something into my rectum!" I was speechless! He explained that his cell door was left open and someone had got in two nights prior and put something in his rectum while he was sleeping.

He held his arms up to estimate the size of the object; it had measured 12 inches in length. He exclaimed, "I can feel it! It's this big!" I tried to gather my wits after hearing about this horrific event. I offered to perform a visual exam, but he vehemently refused. Charles did have a history of paranoia, according to the psychiatrist's note. He was currently taking Vistaril 50 mg. at bedtime for sleep. He admitted he'd been too sound asleep to wake up when it happened. I asked him why he didn't tell his deputy. He replied, "I didn't want to get them mad at me." He also admitted everything was working okay in the 'going to the bathroom' department. That comment made no sense if he was relating the facts correctly.

As I was trying to figure out how to manage this medical complaint, I realized there were Medical, Mental Health, and Dept. of Corrections components involved. I notified the on-call MD and explained the patient's claims to her. She was extremely concerned by his complaints! The MD ordered the Sergeant to be notified regarding a possible PREA (Prison Rape Elimination Act) incident. The MD ordered the patient to be sent to the ER for X-rays and a referral to Mental Health for follow-up.

The MD added one more tidbit of information that I had never known in the 15 years I had worked at Oakwood Medical. She told me about an incident that had happened recently in a dorm in the protected custody building. Three inmates had developed syphilis while in custody! Science is at the point where the lab could determine that the DNA of the infections was all from the same person! (The MD saw the 1st patient because of a rash. The kind of rash a person develops with untreated syphilis! She didn't elaborate on how the two other patients were diagnosed.)

Charles was taken to the ER. There was an object in his rectum that wasn't radiopaque (meaning it didn't block the x-rays like bone or metal would). He could apparently pass it on his own. But it looked different than stool on the x-ray.

Update: Charles was scheduled to be seen by an MD to obtain cultures to rule out STD. He was a "no show" for the appointment. The case was never fully resolved. We may never know what happened. I never had the time to follow up with Mental Health. But the deputies will check the cameras in the dorm after the sergeant is notified of the possible PREA incident.

The two most important days in your life
are the day you're born
and the day you find out why.

-Mark Twain

The Standoff

A simple knee complaint escalated when the inmate refused to walk downstairs. Deputies gathered; tension rose. He insisted he couldn't move — until paramedics gave him benzodiazepines. Then he cooperated, savoring the attention. He returned hours later with no injury noted. I felt played — and unexpectedly sad. In jail, manipulation often masks loneliness.

It started out like any other call—a report of a simple knee strain. Routine. Or so we thought. But it turned into something unique and much bigger than any of us saw coming.

"Hey, we've got a man down in the minimum area," said my coworker, Linda, glancing up from the computer. "Complaint of knee pain." We quickly checked the computer for his medical history. I nodded, already pulling up his chart. Nothing remarkable stood out.

Linda and I headed to the barracks where the injured inmate was housed. He was upstairs, so we climbed the stairs to the second floor to find him. The deputies responded as well. The call came at the end of custody's day shift. Our doctors had gone for the day.

We were pulling our abbreviated crash cart—with a machine to measure blood pressure, pulse, and temperature, along with a glucometer, oxygen, dressings, emergency meds (aspirin, glucose gel, and meds for diabetic emergencies), a suction machine, and supplies to start an IV; all hauled upstairs with the help of inmate trustees. It's a lot to carry, but there's never any knowing what we'll find when we get to the man down.

When we arrived, the inmates in the barracks instinctively froze on their bunks. They knew the drill: stay out of the way when Medical arrives.

One of the inmates pointed outside. “He’s out there, on the stairs.”

We found him standing at the top of the external stairwell. Mid-to-late 40s, holding onto the railing with a dramatic flair.

“You all right?” I asked, squinting at him against the fading sun.

“No, ma’am,” he said solemnly. “Heard a pop. My right knee's done. Ten outta ten pain.”

I asked if I could lift his pant leg to assess his knee. He agreed. So I bent down and gently lifted his cuff. His knee looked fine. No swelling, no redness. I checked the other one for comparison. His right knee was identical to the left.

“Can you walk with support? We can help you inside,” I offered.

“Absolutely not,” he replied, shaking his head. “Pain's too much.”

Linda and I exchanged a glance. His face didn’t reflect the 10 out of 10 pain he'd reported. And his vital signs were stable; this was confusing because vital signs often change when someone is in a lot of pain. Linda and I had seen many sprained knees and ankles on inmates from playing handball or as a result of an altercation. This patient was claiming the injury had occurred while he was standing still.

“Did you fall?” Linda asked.

“Nope. Just turned to go back in and boom.”

It was nearing the end of the Custody shift, and the deputies were fidgeting. The audience of inmates watching from nearby windows was growing.

“Vitals are stable,” I muttered. “Doesn’t look like anything's wrong.”

“He won't budge,” Linda whispered. “Do we call it?”

I sighed. “Let’s call the ambulance to transport him to the ER.”

The problem was, non-emergencies wait. A long time. When Custody bosses learned the ETA was more than an hour, they overrode our medical decision and called for a Code 3 response. They wanted this man down resolved before the start of the next shift.

"Code 3!" one of the bosses barked into his radio. "Get Fire and Paramedics here now."

Sirens wailed 10 minutes later. The Fire Department and paramedics swarmed the scene, squinting up at us on the platform.

"What's the story here?" one fireman asked.

"Possible sprain," I explained. "Pain, no visible injury, normal vitals. Refusing to move."

Another fireman knelt by the inmate. "Where's it hurt?"

"Right here," he moaned, tapping his knee with exaggerated care. "Unbearable."

"Can you bend it at all?"

"Not a chance."

This inmate was holding two nurses, a dozen of the Day shift deputies, and now the Fire Department hostage on this platform at the top of a flight of stairs in front of many other inmates.

One of the seasoned firemen conferred with their coworkers; they are Advanced Cardiovascular Life Support certified and can give medications according to their protocols.

I heard one of them murmur, "Let's give him a low-dose of IV benzodiazepine. Calm him down so we can move him..."

My eyebrows nearly shot off my face.

"Seriously?" I mouthed to Linda. She just shook her head.

I couldn't believe my eyes; the firemen also looked at the "injured" knee and decided this was the necessary treatment. I was worried the inmate audience would be taking notes on how to get a dose of IV medication and a trip to the ER to try it sometime.

The crowd of inmates watched like it was a performance. The injection was administered. The inmate sighed audibly. Then he allowed himself to be backboarded, splinted, and gently carried down the stairs like royalty to the waiting ambulance.

Two hours later, he strolled back into Oakwood Medical, still with the glazed look of an IV med bolus and ambulating without any difficulty.

"What did the ER say?" I asked.

"Nothing wrong," he replied with a shrug.

The ER doctor had found nothing wrong with the inmate's knee, and no new medications were ordered. I was busy caring for other patients with infected wounds and raging hypertension, but I was still confused thinking about the crazy scenario around this inmate earlier that evening, with him standing outside on the stairs, refusing to move.

No prescriptions, no diagnosis. Just a round-trip ticket to the ER, a bit of IV sedation, and the attention of two nurses, a dozen deputies, half the Fire Department, and every inmate within view.

Back in Medical, I turned to Linda as we unpacked our gear.

"Did we just get played?"

She let out a short laugh. "Like a violin."

We are all trained to be of service to those who need help, but I can't say if we helped this inmate any more than to get a transient high off a dose of IV medication and a trip to the ER. Fortunately, we never had a repeat performance of this patient encounter.

We didn't fix an injury that day. But maybe we treated a different kind of pain—the kind that craves attention in a place where you're often invisible. I felt played—and yet I also felt strangely sad. Sometimes, neediness and manipulation often hide deeper needs that intertwine with loneliness in ways that defy simple judgment.

> ***Tact is the ability to tell someone to go to hell in such a way that they look forward to the trip***
> *- Winston Churchill*

Code for Mom

Some weekends, my phone became a lifeline for frantic families reacting to cryptic calls from inside. Mothers sobbed, brothers demanded answers. Bound by HIPAA, I could say little, yet I carried their fear. One Spanish-speaking family's desperation stayed with me. Some nights, I was the thin thread connecting them to someone they loved.

I had the most interesting weekend talking to several family members of mentally ill young men in their 20s. As Charge Nurse, I answer phone calls. LOTS of phone calls. The number of calls I received on a weekend in April 2017 was something I had never experienced before...

Saturday afternoon started with a mother calling about her son. She was unaware of where he was for a few days and had recently found out he was in jail. She wanted to know what was happening with him, but Oakwood Medical did not have a signed Release of Information that authorized medical staff use to give information about a patient's status to the person identified in the Release. Her son refused to sign the Release of Information because he believed his mother was responsible for putting him in jail. All I could do was assure her the deputies would keep him safe.

I requested a Mental Health visit from Helen, a favorite MH staff member. I told the patient's mother I was putting in a request to have him seen by a member of the MH staff (all of whom are credentialed therapists) to make sure he was housed in a safe location. There were several calls to the mother to explain that the MH staff were going to interview her son. The mother also called to ask for updates on her son. The calls ended with the mother expressing her gratitude for the support (even though I couldn't give her details, just assurance the deputies would keep him safe and MH would see him). She began crying as she hung up the phone. I wasn't far behind.

The next call was from an inmate's brother. He said he had gotten a "collect call" and needed to know what was going on with his brother, who had a mental health diagnosis. The caller was deeply concerned for his brother's safety. The caller also didn't make much sense; I needed more information. Soon the caller sheepishly admitted his phone couldn't actually accept collect calls from jail. Apparently, he had received a collect call request; it was "code" that something might have happened to his brother.

I read the notes in his medical record; he had been seen bending over the upstairs railing in a Lockdown unit the night before, one which houses inmates with MH diagnoses. MH staff were called, and the inmate was rehoused to a single cell on suicide watch, which means the deputy must take a look at the inmate every 15 minutes and document it for the duration of the checks. MH documented that his speech was bizarre, and staff wanted to make sure he was safe.

Two weeks before, another inmate had jumped to his death from the second floor of a dorm in this same Lockdown building. Understandably, the deputies were quite anxious seeing inmates hanging over the railing. The inmate signed a Release of Information so we could tell his brother what was going on with him. I explained the situation to the caller. The caller stated he had visited his brother the previous night, and he kept insisting on knowing more about what was occurring with him. I informed him I was referring him to Mental Health and requested he call back to obtain more information. The brother never called back.

On Sunday, I received a call from a Spanish-speaking woman calling about her 20-something-year-old son with mental health issues housed in Lockdown.

I spoke basic medical Spanish, but my mental health terms were lacking. Fortunately, the woman had her son with her, who could translate. The patient had signed a Release of Information so we could give the mother information about her son. A call had already been made to her from the dorm. It was difficult to ascertain how the information had been relayed to her, but she was concerned for her son's safety because of the call she'd received. There were no recent notes in his medical record written by any discipline. I asked the deputy working in Oakwood Medical if he could call the dorm and ask the deputy to do a welfare check on her son. I also requested a MH visit to check his status. The deputy in the dorm reported back there might have been a threat of bullying, and he would check into it. The medical record showed the patient was taking his meds. All of this information was relayed to the patient's mother.

Later Sunday night, another mother of an inmate in his 30s who'd been arrested the day before wanted to make sure he was getting his prescription eye drops for the corneal ulcer on his eye. We called the pharmacy to clarify the medication, the instructions, and when it was dispensed. The day shift nurses had begun the process and reported to me that they obtained a telephone order for the eye drops to be started immediately for the patient. But it turned out my beloved Medical Center's pharmacy didn't carry the identical medication. I consulted with the pharmacist and then called Oakwood Medical's on-call MD to notify her that the Rx needed to be changed to one in stock. The on-call MD was anxious about getting the Rx initiated. We also needed to clarify that the Rx was in a plastic container. He was using it every four hours, and to keep it on his person it had to be a plastic bottle, not glass. The patient started on the eye drops early that evening. I didn't hear back from the patient's mother until Tuesday night; she was upset because she had spoken to him and he hadn't received his mental health medications yet. Her son was going to court the next day, and she was desperate that he start his meds before court because he'd sounded like he didn't make sense when she spoke to him on the phone. His mother insisted he needed these meds so he could understand what was going on in court. I told his mother I would call him to Oakwood Medical and give him his meds. All of his mental health meds had been ordered two days prior, but no one had notified him. I explained how to get his medication and at what time. His mother called back later and was grateful someone had helped her son. This mother sounded like she was on the brink of crying, too.

Some weekends, my phone might as well have been an extension of a grieving mother's heart. Calls poured in from families—frantic, confused, terrified—after receiving cryptic messages from inside. Mothers sobbed, brothers demanded answers, and entire families hovered on the edge of panic. Bound by HIPAA, I could say so little, yet I held their fear like it was my own. Some nights, I became the only thread connecting them to their loved ones' fragile reality.

All these calls made me wonder if some of these inmates have an agreement to call one another's family to notify them of a change. So many calls in two days with a similar request: to check their family member's safety. We have even had family members call after an inmate was sent to the ER in an ambulance after an altercation. But nursing staff never notifies the family when this happens. While they scream at us over the phone for not giving them any information, they also yell that someone called to say they were hurt and were going to the ER. But of course it is against the law for anyone who is currently incarcerated to have visitors in the ER or the hospital.

We must notify the deputies when we get these calls. The patient may be diverted to another hospital for safety reasons.

"Copy that!" they say. Deputy code for "I understand."

> ***I'd rather regret the things I've done than regret the things I haven't done***
>
> *- Lucille Ball*

WTF???

That week felt surreal. A routine man-down call spiraled into gang intel and a classification investigation. Later, an inmate scaled the minimum-security fence and sprinted toward administration, triggering a facility-wide lockdown as visitors stared in shock. I remember thinking, What universe am I working in? In jail, routine care can quickly turn into a security crisis.

This has been a memorable week! I'm the Charge Nurse, so I'm involved in EVERYTHING!

Tuesday night was wild. It's flu season. We were fighting a battle with Influenza A. The MDs decided to quarantine Barracks 2 in the minimum-security area, which houses 60 men. This seemed to be where the fevers originated. Each time an inmate spiked a fever of 101.2°F, the nurse was ordered to perform a nasopharyngeal swab. In layman's terms, jamming a long Q-tip on a bendable wire through their nose and into their throat to touch a tonsil! This is torture for someone who already feels like sh*t.

The nursing staff had to go out to the quarantined barracks for pill call, temperature checks, and diabetic call four times a day.

THEN...the virus escaped to another Barracks.

Barracks 8 was quarantined. So now, nurses had to do pill call, temperature checks, and diabetic call in two quarantined barracks. This was before the 2019 Covid pandemic, so it was very strange to see deputies and inmates walking around wearing masks. Quarantines were not normal. Several of the nurses got sick.

I spoke to the Supervisor at the downtown Main Jail. "Nobody has the flu!"

Main Jail is an old, closed building with stale air! No open windows to help move the air around...and NO ONE IS SICK? Doesn't make sense.

For now, it seemed the virus was contained in the minimum section of Oakwood. Then it happened: the flu virus traveled to Lockdown. This is a different setting; the inmates are in dorms with one door to the sun deck. Lockdown doesn't have the freedom of movement outside the building that the minimum inmates have. Each time an inmate was found to have a fever of 101.2°F, the nurses were to call the on-call MD for permission to have them transferred to the Infirmary.

After calling for two patients with fevers, the on-call MD was paged for the third one. As soon as he called back, he just ordered us to send the patient to the Infirmary. No time wasted with medical history and symptoms!

Swab and transfer to the Infirmary!

Each transfer to the Infirmary needed to be clarified with the Charge Nurse at the Infirmary to make sure they had a bed available for the impending transfer.

I was SO looking forward to finishing my shift – which I did late after giving Report to the Night shift about all the transfers to the Infirmary earlier that night – so I could leave the building and feed the feral cats.

I then walked out and found one of our cats caught in a trap set for skunks, raccoons, and opossums! I released a little tuxedo kitty named Sammie from the trap and tripped the door so no other animal could get stuck!

These traps were supposed to be checked frequently to make sure any animal caught was safe. This didn't seem to happen. One partner who helps with the cats is part of the Custody staff. I called and relayed to her what happened. The traps were removed that day. Sammie was fine after her ordeal.

BUT...Thursday night was going to be full of even more surprises!

A fight in a Lockdown dorm of gang members resulted in injuries. One of the inmates had to go to the ER for sutures. A fight involving several people usually locks down the facility. The participants of the altercation are separated and placed in holding cells.

The inmates must be cleared by Medical before they can be interviewed by the deputies about what happened. Deputies from all units at Oakwood are expected to respond to an altercation, leaving other dorms/areas unsupervised for a short period. There is no movement: no pill call, no wound care, no diabetic call.

This slowed everyone down!

I found out while I was getting transfer paperwork ready for the inmate who needed sutures that he was interviewed by a Gang Affiliation Classification deputy. This was a specialized Classification team. This particular team has to know who is in the specific gang and each member's standing in the gang.

That was Thursday night!

I had Friday off to relax.

Saturday started normally, as if there is such a thing in a jail setting!

I signed in at the West Gate, had my bag searched by the deputy, and proceeded to Medical. As I entered Medical, there was a 30-something-year-old inmate from the minimum area of Oakwood sitting handcuffed, surrounded by several deputies and a Sergeant.

One of the Day shift nurses exclaimed, "He tried to jump!"

I replied, "Like to kill himself?"

She said, "No.....to escape!"

Apparently, the inmate was arrested Friday night because he disregarded a restraining order against him by his ex-girlfriend. There was a significant amount of methamphetamine, too!

So, on Saturday, he decided he needed to get back to his ex!

He jumped a fence in the minimum area, which has straight "Candlestick" fencing. The rest of Oakwood has double "Candy cane" curvature fencing. He made it over the first fence, then headed west to the Administration building close to the front of the facility.

Walking toward the same gate staff and visitors use when exiting the facility, he is spotted by visitors waiting for visits at 3 PM. He is still in jail clothing, and the visitors realize something is wrong. A radio call goes out from the West Gate deputy, and all hell breaks loose!

No movement was allowed for 30 minutes right after I came through because Oakwood was immediately locked down. There were four 3-11 PM shift nurses plus our Supervisor waiting at the West Gate to report to work. There was no movement allowed for 30 minutes. But nursing staff were allowed to move slowly to Medical.

The inmate incurred a small laceration after being tackled by a pile of deputies. I needed to send him to the ER for sutures after his escapade. I called Control to arrange for a sheriff's car transport–Code 1.

But there was more going on than we were told!

The Code 1 car with the inmate was tailed by a chase car with two deputies with rifles ready, just in case.

An ambush had been planned on the deputies at the ER. Because of the threat, the deputies had their rifles drawn as they forced the handcuffed, leg-chained, drugged-out inmate into the hospital!

I need a nap!

What a week!

> ***When in doubt, throw doubt out and have a little faith.***
> - E.A. Bucchianeri

Giggles and Poop

I picked up an extra shift expecting calm — but maximum-security had other plans. One detoxing woman kept me on edge, while two others' childlike giggles and heart-shaped hand signs cracked open my exhaustion. Later, I advocated for an elderly man in Protective Custody with chronic incontinence — embarrassed and overlooked. Dignity shouldn't depend on age or incarceration. The shift swung from joy to sorrow — the emotional whiplash of correctional nursing.

The assignments for nurses are made weeks ahead of time. Supervisors try to keep nurses in one area for two weeks for continuity of care. In these two weeks, the nurse gets to know the patients, their diagnoses, what meds they take, and any goofballs who try to get sent to Oakwood Medical for frivolous complaints, or better yet, go to the ER, which is the best field trip ever. This can be done by faking chest pain, headaches, or even contractions if the patient is pregnant. Some of my coworkers didn't like the two-week rotations because it made them more accountable. Even with the best-laid plans, things happen: nurses call in sick, and schedules change.

I took an opportunity to work on my day off one Sunday. I assumed I would continue my assignment in the Protective Custody building. Inmates choose Protective Custody for several reasons. Some are in "PC" due to charges (like child molestation; to protect them from other inmates), alternative lifestyles (LGBTQ), medical diagnoses (HIV), fear that someone in jail may hurt them, and advanced age. Many of them are there for a long time while their cases make their way through court. When a "PC" has a medical appointment in Oakwood Medical, every effort must be made to keep them safe around all the other inmates who are there. The color of their clothing lets everyone know they are "PC."

Giggles

When I arrived for my extra shift, I found out the day-shift nurse was working overtime and had first choice for an assignment. They had been working in the Protective Custody building that morning and wanted to stay there. I ended up being assigned to my favorite place—where my max-security female inmates were.

Their charges were very serious, but they had proven they could get along with other inmates, so they could be housed in a dorm setting with single or double cells. I did not know all of their charges, but after spending time with them over the years, I got to know them in a nurse-patient relationship.

As I was finishing up the evening pill call, a deputy stopped me.

"Nurse Nancy, can you check on the detoxing inmate in cell 3C? She's not looking too good," she said.

"Sure thing," I replied, nodding as I pushed my med cart toward the cell.

After completing my assessment and leaving the dorm, two inmates locked in their cell started pounding on the door to get my attention. I was afraid something was wrong, so I turned to see what was going on. The inmates were a fifty-something former nurse and her roommate.

"Nurse Nancy!" they called out in unison, waving their hands frantically.

As I looked at them, I could see they were making the sign of a heart with their hands. I stopped pushing my med cart and made the sign of a heart back at them.

"What's going on, ladies?" I asked, stepping closer to their cell.

They giggled like teenagers.

"Oh, come on now," I said, laughing. "You're making me blush!"

They burst into laughter, and I couldn't help but grin. It was such a small moment, but it reminded me of the human side of this place—a brief escape from the reality of their situations. It made my day to see these ladies, facing life-changing charges, escape their situation for a moment and find joy in a simple interaction.

Ben's Story

After a day off, I was back with the Protective Custody inmates. First, I medically assessed and cleared two inmates involved in an altercation. Then, one of the nicest deputies approached me:

"Hey, Nancy, can I talk to you about Ben?" asked a deputy.

Ben was an 83-year-old man incarcerated for over a year, whom I had seen daily for diabetic call. He was always polite. My coworker Skylar laughed about Ben; she remembered one day when he greeted her with, "Hey, ggguuurrrrlllllllll!!!"

"Sure," I said, pausing to look at the deputy's concerned expression.

"Ben's been having some issues," he began. "He can't control his stool, and the guys in his dorm are getting fed up. They've been helping him, but it's wearing thin."

I checked his medical record to see if his doctor knew about his incontinence. It had in fact been noted as chronic fecal incontinence.

"Yeah, it's in our file for extra clothing," the deputy confirmed. "The thing is, he needs to be moved to a dorm where he can get help. No one's followed through on it yet."

The deputy said he had asked several other nurses to rehouse Ben to a unit where he could get assistance with his ADLs (Activities of Daily Living, which include help with toileting). Several nurses told him they would look into it, but never followed through.

I frowned. "I'll handle it. But you know moving him is going to be hard. He's been here for over a year. This is his 'home.'"

The deputy nodded, "I know. But it's what's best for him. I hate to see the guy struggle like this."

Later that night, I faxed the request for rehousing to Classification. Once the paperwork arrived in Classification, the deputies looked at Ben's file and completed arrangements to move him to the new dorm at Main Jail downtown. As I filled out the paperwork, I pictured Ben packing up his belongings and being loaded into the van.

"Do you think he'll be okay downtown?" I asked the deputy as I handed him the forms.

"It'll be better for him in the long run" he said with a small smile.

I didn't tell Ben about the move—protocol requires us not to. Sometimes, when inmates know ahead of time they are being transferred downtown, they might make calls that could become a safety issue for the transferring deputy. Also, inmates in Ben's dorm might send contraband with him to distribute downtown. It is always safer not to tell an inmate they are being moved to another dorm. Still, I felt a pang of guilt.

This job is always interesting. One day, it's all about giggles; the next, it's about poop and trying to maintain an old man's dignity while in jail. These are the kinds of experiences that creep into my head as I try to fall asleep at night. The range of interactions from dorm to dorm between the men and the women at Oakwood make for opportunities to share a moment in someone's life and provide unique nursing care to custom-fit every situation.

It's a good thing I love a challenge.

> ***If you have the ability to love, love yourself first.***
>
> \- Charles Bukowski

An Easter Surprise

Everything unraveled — heavy assignments, crises, nonstop calls. Then Prinnie admitted she'd swallowed 24 Benadryl, and the shift felt crushing. Grace came in small ways: Chris's steady kindness and a deputy who fed the feral cats for me. By night's end, exhausted, I saw it as an unexpected miracle — kindness blooming in a hard place.

Easter weekend turned out to be my scheduled weekend to work. My kids have grown up, so we have no more Easter egg hunts, parades, or candy baskets.

Staffing happened to be below the minimum. The Charge Nurse gave me my favorite lady's dorms, "A" and "B," PLUS the Level 4 "C" dorm, which are in the same building. This "C" dorm is usually an assignment by itself because it can be problematic and therefore time-consuming. This was going to be a busy night.

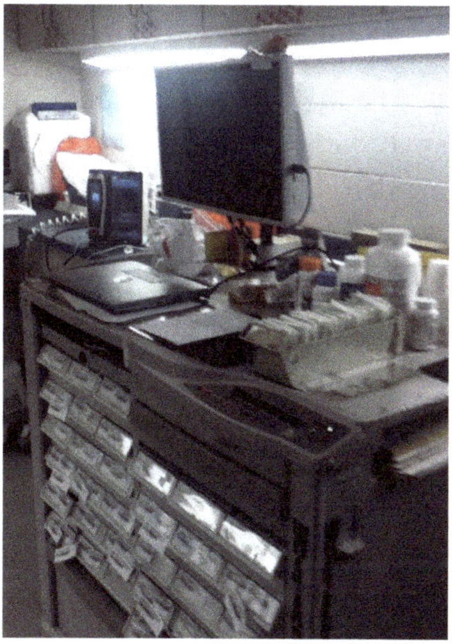

I began my shift trying to log onto the medication cart/computer for the two big dorms: "A" and "B." It wasn't working. I had to go out to check with the Control deputies who were monitoring all the activity in the building and see if I could go into "C" dorm to borrow the medication cart/computer for diabetic call before dinner. Control indicated it was safe to proceed to "C" unit. I gathered my supplies and checked with Control again before proceeding to “A” dorm. This was usually the easy part of my shift. I eventually completed diabetic call in all three dorms and was starting to get my cart ready for the night's pill call. (Having a medication cart/computer that was out of commission meant I had to move all of the medications in the cassettes from “A” and “B” to “C” cart; the medication carts were not interchangeable.)

I heard a tiny knock at the door of the Medical office for “A” and “B” dorms. A member of the Mental Health team was there, someone new I didn’t recognize. She had been speaking with Prinnie, a woman in her twenties with a long, complicated history of trauma, Mental Health issues, and many suicide attempts.

Prinnie admitted she had been hoarding pills in her bra. Nurses giving pills to patients are supposed to watch them swallow their medication to avoid situations like this. Prinnie refused to hand over the pills to the deputies or the mental health staff, so the next step was “use of force.”

WELL...right before the deputies were called (Emergency Response Team in their full riot gear), Prinnie admitted that 90 minutes ago she had taken 24 capsules of Benadryl.

SO...that changed everything!

The MH staff at my door came to tell me Prinnie had admitted to swallowing the 24 Benedryl capsules. This patient was not familiar to me, but I didn’t want to take the time to read her history before meeting with her, as ingesting so many doses of Benadryl was potentially life-threatening.

I got my machine to check her vital signs and proceeded with the MH staff to assess Prinnie. I completed my assessment and informed the deputy in the dorm I would be notifying the on-call MD. The MH staff went to her office to write up the 5150 (a danger to herself).

Prinnie wasn’t excessively sedated from ingesting so much Benadryl, but I needed to go through the motions of handling an ingestion by a patient. Poison Control was notified before calling the on-call MD. The on-call MD knew Prinnie by her reputation for repeated suicide attempts. Medical staff is responsible for the care of a person who has attempted suicide. Mental Health staff documents the need for a 5150 and relocation to the Acute Psychiatric Unit once their medical condition is stabilized.

The Prinnie "mandown" set me back, and cost me my dinner break. (I'd brought some carrots and celery with my dinner that night, so I quickly grabbed them out of my locker. They would be my dinner.) The deputy and I brought Prinnie to Oakwood Medical via wheelchair to be observed until the ambulance arrived to take her to the ER. I gave Report to the Charge Nurse, documented my notes to include details of my interactions with Mental Health and Prinnie, and headed back out for the evening pill call.

Then I gave Control a "heads-up" that I was covering the whole building that night. Control needs to know this information in case of emergencies in the other dorms. I was able to start pill call 15 minutes early, but the Special Management dorm (the ladies with mental health issues) needed me to go door-to-door tonight. When the lower level of cells are completed the second floor cells are opened a couple at a time. It took over two hours to complete pill call and assessments. (Pill call and assessments usually range anywhere from one hour to ninety minutes.)

I proceeded to "B" dorm – my favorite high-security ladies! This would be a piece of cake! No drama, no suicide attempts; just pill call. It was the high point of my night. By this time, I had been on my feet for six hours.

Then I went to "C" dorm. There aren't many patients here. These ladies are kept in single cells within a small dorm. I went inside each dorm, door-to-door, and gave medications through the tray slot. (These inmates couldn't have the doors to their cells opened unless there were several deputies present.)

Halfway through pill call one of my coworkers, who had finished early, was sent over to help me out. She completed pill call in "C" dorm, which allowed me to start all of my documentation for the shift: wound care, blood pressure checks, detox assessments, etc.

At 11:30 p.m., I heard a tiny knock at the door to "A" and "B" dorms' Medical room.

The Mental Health staff member who had been talking in a very kind and gentle voice to Prinnie came back to let me know she had written an email to her supervisor detailing how prompt I was after Prinnie admitted to taking all the Benadryl.

She expressed her gratitude that I had responded in a timely fashion to an urgent, potentially life-threatening situation. I looked at her in total disbelief!

The Mental Health staff didn't usually sing the praises of the nurses. I had to ask the staff member's name; such a caring person. Her name was Chris.

She added that she documented an Incident Report that would be sent to the MDs, psychiatrists, and the pharmacy, saying that the nurse on the Day shift had given Prinnie a pill and she placed the pill on her table. Because of her history of hoarding medication, the nurse should have reported this to the deputies and mental health immediately. This hadn't been done.

Chris seemed to be an extraordinary member of the Mental Health staff. She cared for the inmates and went above and beyond as a rule for anyone who needed help. We headed back to Oakwood Medical after midnight. I told Chris how impressed I was with how much she cared for the inmates.

One of the deputies met us on our way back. The deputy was feeding the feral cats that night; she had heard how busy I was, and happily fed all the cats.

Chris said, "I worked at Oakwood Mental Health in the late 1990s. A woman co-worker took care of the feral cats. Her name was Jelly. I called her when I saw a sick cat one night, and she drove from the Santa Cruz mountains to take care of that cat!"

At this moment, I no longer felt my aching feet. I knew this was my Easter miracle.

Jelly was my good friend who had retired a few years ago. After she retired, I started helping out with feeding and caring for the feral cats. When I told Jelly that Chris was back at Oakwood, she was thrilled to hear the good news.

After the challenging night I'd had, it was like getting a little hug from the Universe, telling me that everything was going to be okay. Such was my Easter surprise.

> ***Be happy for this moment.***
> ***This moment is your life.***
> - Omar Khyyam

MRSA, MRSA, MRSA!

She rushed toward me, shouting about MRSA. Panic swept the dorm. The stigma spread faster than the infection. Her wound was healed, treatment complete — but HIPAA kept me vague as anxiety simmered. Then another woman claimed she couldn't breathe, fear feeding fear. In jail, anxiety is contagious.

One afternoon, as I was trying to complete diabetic call before dinner, Patsy, a 20-something female inmate, walked down the hall from the medium-security dorm, announcing loudly, "I have MRSA and no one is doing anything about it!"

This was in 2017 when these words struck fear in the hearts of anyone hearing them. MRSA (Methicillin-resistant Staphylococcus Aureus) infection is caused by a highly contagious type of staph bacteria that has become resistant to many antibiotics and is therefore known as a superbug. At-risk populations include people who live in crowded conditions. MRSA often begins as a painful skin boil, frequently accompanied by a fever, and is usually spread by skin-to-skin contact.After the COVID-19 pandemic, it remains a significant diagnosis, but doesn't carry the weight it used to because specific MRSA antibiotics have been developed. Treatment typically involves isolation.

These words triggered immediate hysteria among inmates waiting in the hall to have their blood sugar tested (one patient at a time in the Medical office due to HIPAA precautions and safety), trustees delivering dinner trays to the units, and deputies in the dorms.

"Who has MRSA? Oh my god! How can this be happening? I'm going to get sick!" were just some of the comments heard in the hallway and dorms.

I stopped what I was doing to assess Patsy's complaint.

I had her sit in the medical office. I took her vital signs, a routine assessment for any patient. She repeated her complaint. "I have MRSA and no one is doing anything about it!" I asked to see her wound, and she showed me a healed area on her arm: no erythema (redness), no edema (swelling), and no drainage. I looked up her medical record and saw that she had been diagnosed with MRSA several weeks ago and was sent to the Infirmary and isolated per our protocol. Nurses provided wound care. Patsy was given antibiotics. Once she completed them and her wound healed, Patsy returned to her bunk in the medium-security dorm.

I returned to the dorm to explain my findings to the deputies and sergeant without telling anyone about her medical condition (per HIPAA regulations). The diabetics had to wait. MRSA carried a lot of weight in terms of health priorities. Without divulging Patsy's medical history, I informed the sergeant that I had assessed the patient and saw no indicators of an active infection. Still, a culture from drainage is necessary to diagnose an infection as MRSA.

The sergeant needed more information to ensure the dorm would stay "safe." I reinforced the fact that I saw no open wounds on the patient. It didn't help that Patsy continued to yell, "I have MRSA and no one is doing anything about it!" when she went back to her dorm.

Dinner was being served. I had been dealing with this patient's complaint for 45 minutes. The sergeant called the lieutenant to report my findings. The diabetics grew bored and hungry and left to eat dinner; I had to find them and have them sign a Refusal for Medical Services document since they hadn't gotten their blood sugar tested.

The deputies, the sergeant, and the inmates started to calm down. Patsy stopped yelling and started eating. I needed to document the encounter with Patsy, the deputies, and the sergeant. Then I documented each refusal the diabetics signed and their reasons for refusing to get their blood sugars checked. I thought everything was winding down.

THEN, an inmate in the dorm across from Patsy started having difficulty breathing. Deputies called Medical to report the situation. My meal break had to wait. I grabbed my equipment to check vital signs and oxygen saturation and quickly walked to the dorm. The deputies do not encourage staff to run at any time, except when a Medical emergency is announced over the radio.

The patient was a 20-something inmate who was breathing hard. The inmates in her dorm had been moved away, thus she was isolated, so I could safely assess her. Vital signs were fine. Breath sounds were clear. Oxygen saturation was 100%. Her skin was pink and she was oriented to person, place, and time.

Her breathing improved after a few minutes. The sergeant on the unit suggested taking the patient out of the dorm and sitting her where the deputies could keep an eye on her in the deputy's control area. I thought that was a creative way to manage a somewhat chaotic situation.

She was quite upset upon hearing this news. She demanded to be sent to the ER. I explained to the patient and the deputies that her condition looked stable. She insisted on returning to the dorm if she couldn't go to the ER. I told her and the deputies that she must be observed for a period of time after a complaint of difficulty breathing. When I put my equipment back in the Medical office, I checked her medical history. No medical issues had been listed when she was booked three days ago. No allergies. No history of breathing problems.

I was trying to figure out what these two incidents meant when the sergeant came into Medical. We were alone, so there was no risk of an inmate hearing our conversation. She calmly reported that both Patsy and the other inmate were on her radar. The sergeant believed that these inmates were conspiring to go to the ER for some reason; maybe to obtain drugs and bring them back to the dorm.

"Do you know how much time I spent with these inmates? I still have to document all of this!" I tried not to raise my voice with the sergeant.

Deputies interview inmates and know their criminal histories. But the medical staff doesn't know anything about what they have done to end up incarcerated. In any case, I was grateful to the sergeant for her explanation. She assured me her deputies would watch the inmate so I could leave for a meal break. I did not tell her that my meal break was no longer an option.

I left the building and walked by the area where the patient who had difficulty breathing was seated. She looked angry, but had no signs of dyspnea (difficulty breathing). I made sure to tell the deputies to call Medical if her condition worsened.

Moments like that remind me how fragile emotional stability is inside those walls. Anxiety is contagious in jail.

> ***No act of kindness, no matter how small, is ever wasted.***
>
> \- Aesop

Where Is My Pen?

When I realized my pen was missing, my stomach dropped. In jail, a pen can become a weapon. Deputies froze nearly 100 inmates mid-process, the silence turning suffocating. I found it in a rarely used pocket, embarrassment rushing in. The Deputy calmly announced, "The pen has been located," and the room exhaled. He teased me for months, but the lesson stuck: in jail, safety hinges on the smallest details.

Nurses and doctors in medical settings must carry equipment to handle various situations. A stethoscope, pens, tools to measure erythema (redness of a wound) and TB test induration (a bump that develops when someone has a positive reaction), and bandage scissors often fill the pockets of lab coats or scrubs. For staff working in custody settings, misplacing any of these items could lead to life-threatening consequences.

I used a pen to take notes and fill out written documents since we did not have electronic medical records at the time. I always thought I was extremely careful with my equipment—until the night I couldn't find my pen. Losing a pen in a corrections facility is a serious matter. Inmates can turn even a simple pen into a weapon.

My ordeal began on a Friday evening while a coworker and I processed 80-90 weekenders. Low-level offenders were allowed to keep their weekday jobs while serving their sentences on weekends. This arrangement allowed them to arrive at Oakwood on Friday night and leave Sunday afternoon to receive credit for serving their sentence.

The process started around 6 p.m. The weekenders were brought to a large room for medical assessments to ensure they were fit to stay. Each was asked for a brief medical history similar to what is done during Booking: any history of allergies, current prescription medications, any open wounds, suicidal tendencies, prior incarcerations, or substance use that could lead to withdrawal issues in jail. Repeat visitors, familiar with the routine, answered quickly, helping the process move along.

It was a formidable task for two nurses to question 80-90 people in just two hours, take a set of vitals, document current medications, have patients sign a Release of Information to fax to the pharmacy so the inmate could receive their meds during the weekend, and answer their questions.

Weekenders were quietly milling around or seated, depending on the custody staff assigned to process them. After we finished assessments, the deputies took over, explaining the next step: "dressing out" into jail clothing. I was able to get through the task without a glitch many times—until that one night.

While they spoke, I realized my pen was missing. My heart raced as I checked and rechecked my pockets, only to confirm the worst: my pen was gone. I quickly informed Deputy Manasca, who paused to ensure I was certain. When I affirmed my pen was indeed missing, he took a deep breath and addressed the inmates:

"Hold up! One of the nurses is missing a pen. No one goes anywhere until it shows up!"

My heart pounded. The realization that my mistake was delaying nearly 100 people added to my anxiety. As the deputies searched and questioned the inmates, I frantically checked my pockets again. To my embarrassment, I found the pen in a pocket I do not usually use.

Sheepishly, I informed Deputy Manasca, "I found my pen, and I apologize for the inconvenience."

He remained composed, quietly responding, "Thank you." Turning back to the group, he announced, "The pen has been located. Proceed to get dressed out."

For months afterward, I repeated my apologies whenever I saw Deputy Manasca, and he humorously asked if I needed an extra pen. His calm demeanor during such a high-pressure moment left a lasting impression on me. Another deputy might not have been so understanding, and I was deeply grateful for his professionalism.

Working in corrections taught me the importance of vigilance and teamwork. The deputies' efforts to keep civilian staff, inmates, and themselves safe were extraordinary, though the job demands often impacted their health. I was always happy to assist whenever deputies had questions about their medications or appointments.

Safety in jail depends on vigilance in even the smallest things. Thank you to all the custody staff at Oakwood for keeping us safe and for your dedication throughout the years we worked together.

> ***All you need is love.***
>
> \- Paul McCartney

The Apple Intern

He arrived shackled to a gurney, pale and sweating — five days post-op from a perforated appendix. Deputies had mistaken his prescribed pain pills for contraband and booked him, leaving him for days without antibiotics or pain control. A Yale graduate and Apple patent-law intern, he'd been raised with privilege and promise. Jail humbled him fast. I sent him straight to the ER, reminded of how quickly life can unravel — anywhere.

One evening shift, while I was Charge Nurse, a call came in from Lockdown. One of the nurses needed to send an inmate to Medical for observation before transport to the ER. She had four dorms to manage and pill call to complete, and couldn't monitor him closely. Oakwood Medical had one individual room reserved for patients requiring observation, complete with a gurney and near the Medical deputy.

When the inmate arrived, sitting in a wheelchair, he looked miserable—eyes sunken, face taut with pain. We helped him onto the gurney, keeping him as comfortable as possible before the deputy shackled him.

His name was Harrison. Twenty-six years old. Five days post-op from a perforated appendix. He complained of severe abdominal pain. His body was curled inward, arms wrapped around his midsection, his breathing shallow. As I introduced myself and checked his vital signs, he muttered something about "Apple" and "intern." At first, I thought he might be delirious from infection. When I pulled up his medical records, I saw the problem immediately—he was supposed to be on antibiotics and pain medication. He had never received either.

As I spoke with him, he calmed down and started to open up. His family was from Los Angeles—"elitists," he called them. He had graduated from Yale and had landed an internship at Apple, studying patent law. But he hated it. He never explained exactly what landed him in community service, only that he was required to show up every weekend.

The details of his medical crisis unraveled piece by piece. His appendix had ruptured while at work, and he was rushed to Kaiser for emergency surgery. But instead of staying to recover, he left AMA (against medical advice) the very next day—determined to show up for his community service shift. He brought his post-op medications with him. That was his mistake.

Deputies spotted the bottle of pain pills in his pocket. In their eyes, that was possession of opiates. Just like that, he was "rolled up"—community service revoked, booked, and immediately placed in Lockdown. He never had a chance to explain.

For four days, he lay in a crowded dorm with 60 other men, his body fighting infection, his stomach a focus of pain. No one checked on him. No one *knew*. If a nurse in Booking had flagged him—if someone had simply picked up the phone to notify us of an incoming patient with a post-op perforated appendectomy—he wouldn't have gone unnoticed for so long. Even the deputies, usually indifferent, had grown concerned. They noticed Harrison wasn't eating.

As he lay there, shackled to the gurney, Harrison spoke softly, his voice carrying a new weight of understanding. Jail had taught him more in a few days than law school ever had, and none of the lessons were good. He had spent his life in privilege, surrounded by structure and predictability. Now, he was just another inmate—ignored, dismissed, suffering alongside men society had long since abandoned. And there was nothing he could do about it. Maybe, he told me, he would rethink his career path. Maybe patent law wasn't where he belonged after all. I later found out he was treated at the ER, and returned to Oakwood minimum housing.

> ***In order to write about life,***
> ***first you must live it.***
> - Ernest Hemingway

I Have a Blister on my Foot

Mary limped in and peeled back her sock to reveal a severe foot infection. She'd had multiple detox checks, yet no one had looked closely. I tried to send her to the ER, but she was being released—and we "couldn't interfere." Days later, I learned she'd needed IV antibiotics. Relief and frustration collided. In chaos, serious problems are easily missed.

One particular evening, my assignment was medical care in three dorms for female minimum-security inmates. Many of them had jobs in laundry, were janitors in the women's part of the jail, or worked in Dietary, moving food carts to the different units. While I was administering medications during pill call, a woman named Mary limped up to my medication cart. She was a Native American woman in her fifties who was arrested two days ago. She was on the alcohol detox protocol, so before the administration of her dose of Librium, I had her take a seat to check her vital signs and ask questions to determine her orientation or lack thereof.

She approached the chair; one sock was hanging off her right foot. Mary was having great difficulty walking. I helped her to the chair. "I went to court today, but the judge wouldn't release me from custody because I couldn't walk very well," she said. Mary may have heard from a jailhouse attorney that they couldn't release her without treatment, but that was incorrect. I asked to see her foot. She removed her sock, with my help, and what I saw upset me. Her right foot was erythematous (reddened), edematous (swollen), and shiny. It was badly infected. Mary said it had looked like this for a couple of days.

"Did you show your foot to the nurses?" I asked.

"Nobody asked me about it," Mary replied.

I felt frustrated that the nurses who had seen her before me (a nurse saw her every 6-8 hours to assess for alcohol withdrawal and administer medication) never looked at her foot to get her some desperately needed medical care. I decided to have her sent to the ER that night. It was after hours, and calling an on-call MD to describe this infection over the phone didn't seem adequate. She needed an MD to take a good look at it in person.

However, a sudden procedural complication emerged. Just moments after I'd decided to send Mary to the ER, a deputy called out her name. She was being released. I was stuck in an impossible situation. In a previous similar scenario, I'd had support from a sergeant on duty who authorized a newly released inmate to be taken to the ER for a courtesy drop-off because he was confused. I was hoping for the same support for Mary.

But now a different sergeant was doing rounds on the unit (checking the log book, checking for any unusual interactions with inmates, etc). I approached him, explained Mary's infected foot, and asked if she could have a courtesy drop-off at the ER when she was released from custody. His response was abrupt and bureaucratic. He raised his voice and said, "We can't interfere with her release from jail!"

I was horrified.

I quickly explained to Mary that I'd tried to get her a ride to the ER, but couldn't because she was released from custody. I suggested she try to get herself to the ER as soon as possible.

I thought about her after I left work when my shift was over. It really bothered me that I couldn't get her the medical help she needed. A few days later, I spoke with another inmate who knew Mary. She'd made it to the ER and was admitted to the hospital to treat the infection in her foot. She was receiving intravenous antibiotics. I emailed our Medical Director with Mary's information and asked him if there was anything else I could have done. Dr. Sherbakov's answer was, "No. When inmates are released, they are expected to be out of the facility in a certain amount of time."

The story of Mary is more than an isolated incident. It never really stops. The next inmate with a complicated medical problem soon arrived to become my next challenge. This case highlights broader issues within correctional healthcare: Marginalized populations often receive suboptimal medical attention. This suggests that for many incarcerated individuals, detention might represent their most consistent opportunity for good medical care.

> ***You cannot do a kindness too soon,***
> ***for you never know how soon it will be too late***
> \- Ralph Waldo Emerson

Rolled Up from a job in the Laundry

When the familiar laundry trustee appeared in maximum security, I was stunned. She quietly explained she'd refused unsafe, inappropriate expectations placed on the women in laundry — and it had cost her safety and status. In jail, punishment comes swiftly for those who assert boundaries. Listening to her, I felt both admiration and sorrow.

Inmates in minimum security have opportunities to work as Trustees. While the job options aren't exactly equal between men and women – which makes sense since there are fewer female inmates – the ladies still have some decent job choices. Female inmates can work as janitors, help distribute meals, or tackle laundry duties. But getting these jobs isn't just a free-for-all; important health checks are involved...

Before an inmate can start working, they've got to be cleared by Medical. This means no open wounds, no illnesses that would interfere with job performance, and they need a negative TB skin test. It's pretty straightforward. When inmates get jobs, staff is super careful about tracking their movements; they sign in and out on a whiteboard so the deputies always know exactly where they are. Most inmates will tell you that having a job helps the time pass much faster.

One evening, while preparing for pill call in the maximum-security dorm, I spotted an inmate I recognized from the Trustee dorm. I'd seen her before in minimum security, and she'd always been friendly and respectful. Now she was dressed out in max security clothing.

Inmates sometimes get "rolled up" from medium security housing for misbehavior and placed in max dorm as a disciplinary measure. But this didn't seem like a typical situation. When she approached my pill call cart, I couldn't help but ask, "What are you doing here?" I'm not usually that nosy, but I had a rapport with her so I felt comfortable enough to say something.

Her response was eye-opening: "I refused to work in the Laundry, so I was placed on 'disciplinary' in max dorm for 30 days," she explained. And then she shared something that was honestly shocking...

She described the condition of the laundry – and trust me, it was way more complex than just washing dirty sheets. "When the dirty laundry arrives, there are sheets that have been fashioned into sex toys," she said. "They leave everything intact when switching out sheets, and it's so disgusting. It made me physically sick."

After a couple days of dealing with these stomach-turning laundry conditions, she knew she couldn't continue. She reported to the deputy that she could no longer handle the job because it was making her ill. The result? Thirty days in max dorm housing, where inmates are mostly confined to their cells and spend time alone.

"I really don't mind," she told me. "I'm just happy to be away from that laundry job. I don't mind being alone."

Her story was genuinely disturbing. While I understood that there are consequences for not completing assigned work, the job conditions she described seemed almost inhumane. Most people think doing laundry is just about throwing bedding in a washer, but clearly, there's so much more going on behind the scenes.

I knew that intimacy happens in jail; that wasn't a surprise. But the idea of a laundry worker having to handle bedding that's been deliberately transformed into sex toys? That's a whole different level of uncomfortable. Some inmates are so careful about cleanliness that they even wash their underwear separately to ensure they're truly clean.

The good news? After her disciplinary period, she was reassigned to a janitorial job and was thrilled about it. When I saw her later, she was genuinely happy in her new role.

This experience was a real eye-opener. It showed me that jail jobs aren't just about keeping inmates busy; they're complex environments with unique challenges. While the system tries to provide meaningful work and structure, sometimes the reality can be pretty complicated.

The inmate's resilience was remarkable. Despite the gross working conditions and the disciplinary consequences, she remained positive and saw her reassignment as an opportunity. It's a reminder that attitude can make a huge difference, even under challenging circumstances.

Her story also highlights the importance of workplace safety and dignity, even in a correctional setting. No worker should feel physically ill or traumatized by their assigned tasks, regardless of their current living situation.

> ***We love the things we love for what they are.***
> - Robert Frost

Girls Just Want to Have Fun .... on the Acute Psychiatric Unit!

Three notorious high-security women hatched a chilling plan: stage simultaneous emergencies to reunite in the acute psych unit. Rochelle feigned suicidal ideation; Lana tied sheets around her neck; Rena blocked her door and attempted self-strangulation. When deputies cut Lana down, my blood ran cold. Only later did we learn it was coordinated — dangerous and manipulative, yet rooted in a longing for connection. It left me shaken, a reminder of how loneliness and confinement can blur the line between desperation and tragedy.

A quick note to say this story really happened. If my former coworkers are reading this, they will know exactly who these inmates are despite me having changed their names. These ladies were on the Level 4 unit, in separate single cells, in separate dorms. They were all well-known to the Medical, custody, and Mental Health (MH) staff. This story had all of us scratching our heads...

The story involves three inmates who had been in custody for more than a year. The first patient was Rena, a twenty-something woman who had asthma, chronic abdominal pain, and mental health issues. Rena had had many encounters with Medical for her asthma problems and stomach complaints. She had also complained many, many times about wanting to kill herself, resulting in many Mental Health encounters. Rena could also "read" staff and knew who she could manipulate.

I was in the MH office one evening when a deputy called from her housing to report that Rena was complaining of feeling suicidal. This complaint automatically generates a protocol where the deputies move the inmate to an area where they can see her and she can't hurt herself while they await MH staff. These inmates spend 23 hours/day in their cells, so these events make for extra time out of them, in addition to their regular daily hour of "program time," when they can make phone calls, take a shower, and watch TV. The MH staff on duty knew the call was code for "please bring me a book!" But they headed out to the dorm to evaluate Rena for her complaints to the deputies.

The next patient was Rochelle, another inmate in her twenties who had not had many medical complaints since the birth of her child the year before. Rochelle did have a relationship with Mental Health, though, due to many complaints of feeling suicidal. She and Rena had developed a relationship while housed in the max security, one which was quite tumultuous at times.

Lana was the third patient. Lana was new to the relationship with Rena and Rochelle. I was not aware of her relationship with MH before this time. These patients are all housed in single cells in different dorms: they have no physical contact with each other or any other inmates. But they can be seen using American Sign Language to communicate during the day. No communication is allowed between them, so they have to wait until the deputies are distracted to do so.

That week, these patients made a pact to go to the Acute Psychiatric Unit downtown so they could be together. They wouldn't actually be together in the psychiatric unit, but there is more of a chance to be physically closer there.

Rochelle convinced one of the MH staff that she was suicidal, and was therefore transferred to the psychiatric unit after a 5150 was completed.

Lana decided to engage in potentially deadly behavior to try to get herself to the agreed-upon destination. The deputy was doing her "rounds" when she found Lana in her cell choking, with bedsheets around her neck. It took a couple of minutes to bring an instrument to cut the cloth off Lana. She was immediately transported to the ER to determine if there was any injury to her airway during this event. Another 5150 was completed. The transporting deputies were instructed to take her to the Acute Psychiatric Unit after she was cleared in the ER.

Rena was the last one to go to the psychiatric unit that day. Rena also undertook dangerous behavior: blocking her cell door with the mattress, making it difficult to open the door. The deputy found her inside, with bedsheets wrapped around her throat. Rena was nonresponsive when the deputies got to her. The ER report documented one-minute intervals of no respiration. I responded to this man-down. Rena was awake when I arrived. We'd had a history of many interactions over the years. With a look of fear in her eyes I had never seen before, she said to me, "I almost died." I nodded. MH documented the 5150. The transporting deputy was told to reroute Rena to the Acute Psychiatric Unit after the ER. Both Lana and Rena had required a Code 3 to be called. The Fire Department and paramedics responded accordingly.

These events are individually not that unusual. But the idea that this was a premeditated collaboration by these patients was horrifying! Rena and Lana believed the only way to reach their goal of being together in the psychiatric unit was to engage in high-risk behavior. Both of these events came dangerously close to tragedies. But the highly skilled deputies on duty likely prevented two in-custody deaths.

It left me shaken, pondering how loneliness and confinement can push people beyond imagination, and how thin the line can be between desperation and tragedy.

> ***Let us literally live from moment to moment.***
> \- Mahatma Gandhi

Who Are You?

A deputy rushed in talking about an inmate reporting sudden arm numbness, trailed by a woman we assumed was Mental Health — until she announced she was the inmate's attorney. The air shifted as she hovered throughout the exam. When we learned he had a rare cerebrovascular condition, the tension sharpened. Her attempt to follow procedures blurred boundaries. In jail, roles matter — and when they blur, so does safety.

I was working one evening at the Oakwood Medical front desk. It had started like any other shift, but then everything went off script. A deputy and a woman sporting a bright yellow visitor's badge rushed an Asian-American inmate in his fifties to Medical.

"I was interviewing him, and he complained that his arms were numb. I got the deputy to bring him right to Medical," the woman said. My coworker June and I looked at each other. We did not recognize the woman. A yellow badge? At first, I thought, *New Mental Health staff, perhaps?*

June began interviewing the patient, including his health history. He had turned in a sick call slip that morning, requesting treatment for athlete's foot. He never said a word about weakness in his bilateral upper extremities. He admitted the continuous numbness in both arms was related to his diagnosis of Moyamoya, which had never been documented in the booking health questionnaire. Moyamoya is a rare blood vessel disorder in which the carotid artery that supplies blood to the brain becomes blocked. Asian heritage increases the risk of developing this disease. Complications include seizures, vision problems, and paralysis associated with strokes.

"I realize that we're used to surprises here, but this one had me second-guessing everything," I told June.

"Exactly!" June replied. "Here we were, thinking we were dealing with a simple foot issue, and suddenly we're facing an entirely different medical puzzle." Then came the moment that left us completely flabbergasted...

The woman who came in with the patient stayed to listen to June's interview. June asked the woman who she was. "I'm his attorney," she coolly replied. June and I looked at each other in complete disbelief. We'd never had an attorney with their client in the Medical department. Usually, all communications with attorneys happen over the phone. And the patient didn't seem to be in any distress. But we had the patient sign a Release of Information so we could legally talk to her.

June left the Oakwood Medical area to call the on-call MD and give a report on this patient and his medical history. The MD authorized sending the patient to the ER. June was careful that neither the patient nor the attorney could hear the details of the arrangements to send the patient to the ER, as a matter of safety for the transporting deputy.

"You are being sent to the ER and will remain in Oakwood Medical until you leave," June told the inmate.

The conversation took another twist when the attorney asked how she could visit him in the ER. The deputy told her she had to speak with the Department of Corrections Captain for authorization. As soon as she heard that, she dashed off, because she couldn't accompany him to the ER after all. In an instant, she was gone, leaving us with a flurry of unanswered questions and an eerie silence hanging in the air.

I kept replaying the events in my head, wondering what it all meant. Who was that woman? How did she manage to catch us off guard in such a critical moment? Why was an attorney allowed into the Medical Department?

It felt like the roles we thought we knew were completely upended. It was one of those surreal experiences that leaves you both intrigued and unsettled—a reminder that behind every face there might be an untold story waiting to challenge everything you thought you knew.

Tonight, the ordinary became extraordinary, and it taught us that in this line of work, surprises are not just possible—they're inevitable.

> ***Always let your conscience be your guide.***
> - Jiminy Cricket

Mr. Lewis and Ryan – A Night in Men's Lockdown

That night was a perfect storm. Lewis came in, on a suicidal concern. Then Ryan, a new booking, spiraled into severe withdrawal — rigid, drooling, his COWS score climbing high after incomplete charting hid how sick he was. I called the doctor, secured orders, and rushed his transfer. Before I could breathe, another inmate claimed an overdose. It was nonstop triage — the raw intensity of jail nursing.

It was shaping up to be just another routine evening in Lockdown. My plan was simple: start pill call in dorms "C" and "D," keep things moving, and maybe, just maybe, finish on time. But, as is often the case in the world of correctional healthcare, the night had other plans...

Back-to-back calls hit me like a one-two punch. The first was from a woman who introduced herself as Mr. Lewis's girlfriend. Her voice was tight with worry—she said they'd just spoken on the phone, and during the call, he confessed he was feeling suicidal. I had no time to process that before the second call came in, this one from a deputy stationed in another dorm. An inmate there was described as lethargic and drooling—classic signs of something going very wrong.

Both situations screamed *urgent.* I didn't waste a second.

First stop: Mr. Lewis. I found him in his dorm and immediately brought the situation to the attention of the deputies. I approached, took his vitals, and gently informed him that his girlfriend had reached out, concerned for his safety. His reaction? A mix of frustration and fatigue. "I'm not suicidal," he insisted. "I was just mad at her." He sounded more annoyed than anything else, but in this line of work, you never take chances. I let him know he'd be referred to Mental Health for a proper evaluation—better safe than sorry.

Then I went to see Ryan. He'd been pulled from his bunk and placed in a holding cell. Only 25 years old and fresh to the system, he'd been booked four days earlier. At intake, he'd told the nurse that he had been using fentanyl and Xanax. Red flags should have started waving during booking.

The Clinical Opiate Withdrawal Scale (COWS) was initiated, and a urine toxicology test had been ordered when he was booked. The COWS assessments done once a day assessed inmates on withdrawal symptoms of nausea/vomiting, stomach cramps, pins/needles, diarrhea, etc., and had scored him mostly 0, with one nurse giving a score of 1. It was as if his detox had been overlooked. But patients detoxing from opiates can receive meds to help with diarrhea, stomach cramps, and insomnia. The detox from Xanax should have been treated like a detox from alcohol. Detoxing from a benzodiazepine can cause severe symptoms.

But here's where things started slipping through the cracks: the urine test was never collected. This wasn't just a simple oversight. Opiate detox is tough, sure—but detoxing from Xanax? That's a whole other beast. It can be downright dangerous—life-threatening, even. If that urine tox screen had been done and showed Xanax and fentanyl in his system, we would have kicked into a higher gear a lot sooner.

When I saw Ryan, he was curled up in a fetal position, arms tucked inside his sleeves like he was trying to disappear. Four days on that bunk. Miserable. Withdrawn—literally and figuratively. I sat down with him and reassessed using COWS: he scored a 13. That's a moderate withdrawal—definitely bad enough to need intervention. He told me he'd never been in jail before. He was in over his head and spiraling.

I moved to the office, picked up the phone, and called Dr. Sherbakov to explain the patient's medical condition. The doctor authorized Ryan's transfer to the downtown Infirmary, where he could finally begin the Suboxone protocol for opiate withdrawal and start a

Librium taper to manage the Xanax detox. For the first time in four days, Ryan had a path forward—he was finally going to get the help he needed.

Later that night, just when I thought things might settle, I walked in on a coworker tending to an infected wound. It looked bad—reddened and edematous. I mentioned the patient probably needed antibiotics, but the nurse brushed it off, clearly eager to end her shift on time. She made no call to the on-call MD.

Meanwhile, I found myself on the phone again. This time, it was Poison Control. Over the months, we'd gotten to know each other quite well. Whenever someone ingests something they shouldn't—foreign objects, pills, cleaning supplies—a nurse calls Poison Control first. That night, a cellmate reported that his "cellie" had swallowed an entire week's worth of meds: Strattera, Remeron, and Risperdal. No one had seen it happen, but that didn't mean we could ignore it. I called the on-call MD, and the inmate was sent to the ER—just in case.

All in all, it was a typical night in Lockdown. You go in expecting to hand out pills and do scheduled assessments. You end up dealing with everything from mental health crises to dangerous detoxes and medication overdoses. It's unpredictable. It's exhausting. And yet, every now and then, you walk away knowing you made a difference.

That night, I helped Ryan. Right place. Right time.

> ***Be the change that you wish to see in the world.***
> -Mahatma Gandhi

Sending Their Love on a Poster

As condos rose around Oakwood, families taped glittered posters to the concrete wall — "We miss you, Dad." Inside, inmates pressed to the narrow windows, searching for color. When they spotted those signs, their faces lit up. Against gray stone, the posters fluttered like small explosions of love — proof someone still claimed them.

Oakwood Correctional Facility has been around for as long as most people in town can remember. Before it housed inmates, it was an almshouse—a last refuge for the poor and forgotten. Over the years, its purpose changed, the buildings were restructured and the grounds secured, until it became the correctional facility it is today.

I remember when Oakwood was surrounded by nothing but dry fields and scrub brush. You'd see rabbits darting across the road at dusk, and occasionally a pair of burrowing owls standing sentinel by the parking lot gates. They had this almost comical way of staring you down—tilting their heads as if trying to understand what you were doing on their land.

"Did you see the owls this morning?" one of the officers once asked as we passed in the hallway.

"Yeah," I replied, smiling. "They were watching me like I was the one behind bars."

He chuckled. "They're probably wondering what we did to get stuck here."

Those days feel distant now. The fields have vanished, replaced first by two massive car dealerships, and then—almost overnight it seemed—by rows of modern condos. Glass balconies. Stainless steel appliances. HOA newsletters.

The wildlife faded. The owls stopped coming. The rabbits disappeared. And suddenly, Oakwood had neighbors—lots of them.

A 12-foot-high wall went up along the north side of the facility, where the condo development pressed closest. The developers tried to make the wall less foreboding. They planted climbing vines and flowering shrubs, and even installed a small walking path behind it for the residents. It worked, in a way. People still bought the units.

"I can't believe people are paying half a million to live across from a prison," my coworker Carla said one morning, sipping her coffee in the break room.

I shrugged. "I guess a good paint job and some landscaping go a long way."

She laughed. "Out of sight, out of mind—until they hear the yard alarms go off."

The layout of Oakwood means that several housing units—two from Lockdown and one of the women's—back right up to that northern wall. From certain angles, if you're standing on the path behind the condos, you can see the outlines of the cell windows through the bar-slatted coverings. I always found it a little surreal—how close those two worlds were. Feet apart, yet divided by a wall, wire, and circumstance.

Visiting hours at Oakwood are rigid. Each unit gets specific days. Holidays are a gamble—if your loved one's unit doesn't have visitation on that day, there's no exception.

That's when I started noticing the posters on the condo development wall.

The first one I saw was on Valentine's Day. I caught a splash of red on the wall. As I slowed down, I saw a giant heart made of construction paper, with glitter catching the sun.

"Happy Valentine's, Tyrell. We Love You Always. –Mom & Jazz"

It stopped me. Not just the sign, but the quiet courage of it. Someone had come out here, probably in the middle of the night or just before dawn, to tape that message to a cold concrete wall. They'd figured out how to make it stick. Maybe duct tape. Maybe command strips. It stayed up for two whole days before the wind took it down.

"I saw your Valentine's poster," I told one of the inmates during a programming session later that week.

He looked up, startled. "You did?"

"Yeah," I said. "It was really sweet. That must've meant a lot."

He nodded, his voice low. "It did. My little sister made it. She said she wanted me to feel remembered."

After that, I noticed more. Christmas. Birthdays. Mother's Day. Even one for a young woman that read, "Congrats on your GED, Destiny! We're proud of you!"

Each poster was a story. A quiet declaration of love. They didn't shout or protest or break rules. They simply said: *You matter to someone.*

Carla once saw one being put up when she drove by early on a Sunday.

"There was a woman standing on a stepladder, taping up a sign," she told me. "She had two little kids with her, holding the corners. Like it was the most normal thing in the world."

I imagined that scene. A quiet morning, the rustle of leaves, the kids trying to keep the poster from folding in the wind. A mother stretching on tiptoe to secure a message of hope.

The candy cane fences around Oakwood are lined with sensors. If anyone tried to get too close or tamper with them, it would set off an alert. So the wall was the only place where these families could send a message, no matter how fleeting.

Some of the posters were decorated like school projects—bright markers, cartoon stickers, photos cut from old albums. Others were just big sheets of cardboard with Sharpie-written words in all caps. But every one of them said the same thing in their own way:

We see you. We haven't forgotten you.

Watching inmates light up when they spotted these colorful reminders from loved ones moved me deeply. Those posters, fluttering in the morning breeze, felt like little explosions of love against gray stone—a reminder that someone out there still claimed them.

And in a place like Oakwood, where time moves slowly and days blur together, I imagine that a poster on a wall—a flash of color in a sea of gray—can mean everything.

> ***You never fail until you stop trying***
> - Albert Einstein

The Night My Favorite Dorm Lost Control

I always felt safe in that quiet women's dorm — until a 19-year-old began violently withdrawing. She convulsed, vomit splattered, and panic spread as inmates screamed and pounded on doors. When the Code-3 sounded and the Emergency Response Team stormed in, the unit shook. Hours later, I finished pill call with trembling hands. Even the calmest places can turn dangerous in a heartbeat.

It was a quiet September evening, the kind that lulls you into thinking the shift might pass uneventfully. At approximately 10 PM, a 19-year-old woman who'd been booked the previous day was out walking in the maximum-security dorm. New bookings are usually out of their cells alone until Classification can determine if they can be safe around others. Classification looks up the inmate's history to determine if there are any "keep aways": inmates they have fought with in previous bookings.

The nurse had just finished pill call in Dorm 2 when the radio crackled in her ear. "Dorm 1 reports inmate nausea. Unsteady gait. Vomiting. Possible detox," came the voice over the radio.

The nurse sighed, looked up her medical history, and headed over. Max security was her favorite dorm. The women there, though tough, were usually cooperative and respectful. The nurse knew most of them by name, or at least by nickname.

When the nurse walked into the dorm, she saw her—the new girl, maybe 19, skinny as a rail with blotchy skin and vacant eyes—pacing in slow circles by the common area. The patient was vomiting into a garbage can. She was detoxing from excessive multiple drug use. The inmate clutched her stomach, then leaned over the garbage can and continued vomiting violently.

"Hey," the nurse called gently. "Let's get you seated, okay?" She didn't respond. Her eyes fluttered. The nurse approached slowly. "You hear me? Are you coming off something?"

She looked up and whispered, "Everything. I was on everything."

From behind their heavy metal doors, the other inmates had seen it all. Looking on, they began yelling and banging on the doors of their cells to demand medical care for their fellow inmate.

"Somebody help her!" a voice screamed. "She's dying, do something!" another yelled.

Within seconds, the chaos intensified. Plastic tubs, books, and fists pounded against reinforced doors. Yelling and screams bounced off the concrete walls.

Then, with a sudden shudder, she collapsed.

The nurse asked the deputy to call for help. "Code 3 medical emergency—Max security dorm. One patient is breathing, but unresponsive. Possible multiple drug detox. Fire response needed immediately!"

Firefighters were on site within minutes. As they rushed in, the nurse in the unit attempted to give a report about the history of the incident:

"She's 19, booked yesterday, and appears to be detoxing from multiple substances. Vomited, collapsed, barely responsive."

"Vitals?" one of them asked.

"I haven't been able to get a full set. The noise—"

The firefighters attempted to assess the patient by hooking up a portable EKG. They couldn't hear each other or hear the patient respond to their questions over the inmates pounding the doors and yelling.

"I can't hear her," the firefighter shouted to his teammate. "We need to move!"

They gently slid her onto a blanket and began dragging her toward the rear sally port, away from the banging, to a quieter location.

They turned as another violent slam rattled the windows. The banging on the cell doors and windows became more violent because the inmates thought the Fire Department was hurting the patient.

That's when it got worse.

From their cells, the other inmates couldn't see clearly. One screamed, "They're hurting her!"

"No! Stop! Don't drag her like that!"

The banging intensified. Doors shook on their hinges. Windows reverberated under the force of the commotion.

The nurse backed against the wall, heart pounding. She stayed in the dorm in case any of the locked-down inmates had injuries.

"Keep calm," she muttered to herself. "They're scared. That's all. They're scared."

The ambulance with the paramedics arrived just in time. They placed the patient on a gurney and rushed them to the ER.

The nurse barely had time to breathe before the sergeant arrived, face tense.

"Lock it down!" she barked, initiating a facility lockdown. An announcement blared over the radio: "Facility lockdown now in effect."

Minutes later, the Emergency Response Team flooded in—full riot gear, helmets, shields, batons. The nurse stood aside as they restored order, moving with trained precision through the dorm.

Once the dorm was secure, deputies inspected the damage. One radioed in, "Broken window panel in Cell 7. Door on Cell 3 won't re-lock. We need to relocate these inmates."

The count took another hour. Every inmate accounted for. No injuries beyond the original patient. Still, the air felt heavy. The whole place had changed in just thirty minutes. Once the dorm was secure, the facility lockdown was lifted.

By the time the nurse finally sat down back in Medical, it was 11:30 p.m., nearly time to go home.

Her hands were still shaking when the phone rang. "Oakwood Medical," she answered tiredly.

"Hey, the dorm's secure now. Can you go back and finish pill call?"

She stared blankly at the wall. "I'm sorry?" she asked.

"Yeah," the deputy said, casual as ever, "some of the inmates insisted they didn't get their meds prior to the medical emergency. The Supervisor says pill call still has to be done."

"But… I mean…" she hesitated, still hearing the banging in her head.

The charge nurse next to her narrowed her eyes and mouthed, *Are you serious?*

The nurse repeated into the phone, "It's almost midnight. We just had a riot."

"Understood," the deputy said. "But the meds still need to be passed."

The Charge Nurse called the supervisor; the supervisor also insisted the evening shift nurse resume pill call.

She exhaled slowly. "I'll go." As she gathered her things, one of the deputies from earlier walked past.

"Hell of a night, huh?" he said.

"Yeah," she muttered, "they've never acted like that before."

He looked back toward the dorm and shook his head. "I can't figure out what set them off. That dorm's usually chill." It had been a long, somewhat terrifying event. None of the deputies could figure out why the inmates responded this violently; it was quite unusual for this dorm.

The nurse didn't answer. Maybe it was fear. Perhaps it was the sight of a young girl slipping toward death. Maybe it was the echo of their own trauma playing out in front of them.

All the nurse knew was that her favorite dorm—the one that always felt safe—suddenly wasn't.

***

As I write and reread this story, it occurs to me that *I* was the nurse in the dorm that night. I remember feeling afraid when I responded to the mandown after the inmate collapsed. The cacophony created by the inmates banging on their doors was deafening. I had been in this dorm many times and had never seen these inmates react in this manner. That night forced me to accept that even the calmest places can turn dangerous in a heartbeat.

Writing in the third person might have been my attempt to look at it from a distance without feeling my fear, the most I ever felt while working at Oakwood.

> ***Expect the unexpected and be ready to zigzag through whatever comes your way***
> -John Cena, professional wrestler

Too Many Burpees Can Hurt You

An inmate told me he'd been forced to do 900 burpees as punishment. Beneath his bravado was fear. Dark urine and flank pain signaled rhabdomyolysis. A urine dip confirmed it, and I called a Code-3. He spent three days in the ICU from a workout meant to "build discipline." Extreme demands can turn life-threatening fast.

One evening, while I was the Charge Nurse, a 20-something, minimum-security male inmate came to Medical complaining of back pain. I had him sit down, and I checked his vital signs. As I assessed him, I asked when his back had started hurting and about the quality and intensity of the pain.

Many minimum-security inmates spend their free time exercising outside their barracks, as the facility lacks a gym. They often use milk cartons filled with water as makeshift weights.

He mentioned that earlier in the day, he had been in a class in the Reentry Correction Program (RCP). During the class, one inmate could not recite all 12 steps of their program, so the instructor forced the entire class to drop and perform 900 burpees. Burpees consist of two movements: a push-up followed by a leap into the air. RCP is a multi-step program that offers classes on job readiness, substance abuse, trauma recovery, and other rehabilitative topics. It is a collaborative effort involving the Sheriff's Department, the Courts, Adult Education, and the Department of Probation.

The patient, who had no significant medical history, clarified that the pain was not actually in his back but in his right flank, near his kidney. Concerned, I asked if he had noticed any changes in his urine color since the pain began. He hesitated before mentioning that his urine had looked a little brown. I tested his urine specimen for the presence of blood; blood was present.

His symptoms were alarming. Intense physical exertion can lead to skeletal muscle breakdown, with muscle tissue fragments potentially clogging the kidneys and leading to kidney failure. This condition, known as rhabdomyolysis, is a medical emergency. Recognizing the urgency, I immediately notified the on-call physician and obtained an MD telephone order to send the patient Code 3 (emergency Fire Department and ambulance response) to the ER. He was admitted to the Intensive Care Unit, where he remained for three days until his lab results normalized and he was discharged. I later emailed my supervisor, detailing the patient's account of the incident. I don't know if my report resulted in any changes. But it made me reflect on how easily extreme physical demands can push vulnerable people into life-threatening conditions.

While researching the RCP program for this story, I recalled my interactions with the women's RCP members. I often walked through the area where the women's RCP participants performed their daily flag-lowering ceremony. Approximately 12-16 women would line up in formation, lower the flag, and fold it with precision. Though not listed as an official part of the program, both men and women RCP members practiced marching drills, complete with a cadence caller leading the routines. At the end of their training, they would compete against each other for the best overall marching performance.

One year, shortly before Halloween (my favorite holiday), I spoke with the women's group. Remembering how my dance instructors had us practice Michael Jackson's "Thriller" routine around this time, I playfully suggested that the cadence caller incorporate some MJ moves into their routine. Though they didn't win the competition that year, rumors circulated that the men's group had enlisted a choreographer who infused their routine with professional touches, ultimately helping them to steal the show.

> ***I dream things that never were and say why not.***
> -George Bernard Shaw

Nelly

Survival can seem random behind bars. One woman jumps over a railing and dies; another keeps finding her way back to breath. Destiny in jail is unpredictable and brutally unequal —some survive, and others, despite support, do not.

One day, I was talking on the phone to Jelly, a former coworker who'd retired from Mental Health at Oakwood. She shared the story of a beautiful woman who had been jailed multiple times there due to her drug addiction. The woman had been housed in the maximum-security single-cell dorm on the second floor. Tragically, one day, to everyone's shock, she jumped over the railing, fell 20 feet, hit her head, and died. The deputies and Medical/MH staff were deeply traumatized by her suicide. As a result, fencing was added to the second floor of this dorm to prevent similar incidents.

This sad story reminded me of another inmate in a similar situation, but with a very different outcome...

Nelly was a beautiful woman in her thirties, housed in medium-security housing. Unlike the maximum-security dorm, this dorm had no fencing on the second floor. The dorm was designed with bunk beds in each "pod" and two floors to house up to 60 inmates. These women were recently incarcerated and adjusting to jail life, often with a lot more drama than the maximum-security inmates. And these inmates had proven their ability to get along with others, which allowed them to live in a dorm setting. They were encouraged to participate in classes to stay occupied.

Whenever I was assigned to work there, I prepared myself for the mindset of "anything could happen tonight." Most nurses preferred any other assignment over working with these women.

One nurse, assigned to Nelly's dorm during a particular shift, recounted the following story:

Nelly was always friendly and respectful with the nursing staff, but clearly had an agenda. She was drug-seeking, trying to convince the Medical staff to give her opiates. She frequently complained of dental problems, back pain, and abdominal pain. Over time, all the medical doctors became familiar with Nelly due to her frequent appointments for vague complaints. The injuries she reported were usually unwitnessed. While Nelly occasionally convinced a few nurses to send her to the ER after hours, the ER staff quickly caught on. Initially, they would order a few doses of opiates, but the doctors reviewing her records in the morning would usually prescribe NSAIDs instead. Eventually, all Oakwood and ER staff were on the same page, and Nelly could no longer obtain opiates from any medical provider.

Determined, Nelly devised a plan no one could dismiss as fake. She went to the dorm's second floor and jumped over the railing, falling 20 feet. She landed on both feet, resulting in compound fractures to both ankles and feet. When the nurse assigned to her dorm responded to the "man down," the first thing Nelly said to her was, "Now I'm going to get some drugs!"

Nelly was transported to the ER, where she underwent multiple surgeries and weeks of physical therapy to walk again. She returned to the Infirmary with a cast and hardware, remaining there until she became ambulatory. From then on, Nelly required orthopedic shoes for the rest of her life.

A few years later, Nelly reappeared at Oakwood in a Special Management dorm with single/double cells and a second floor, but no fencing. New deputies had been hired, and I warned them of her previous jump. The deputy promptly informed the sergeant, who ensured Nelly's movements were monitored closely and that she was never allowed upstairs. Nelly complied with the rules and behaved well.

More years passed, and Nelly again returned to Oakwood, now in her early fifties. She was still beautiful, now with striking white hair.

This time, she was placed in the maximum-security dorm, which also lacked fencing on the second floor. I once again reminded the deputy about Nelly's history. Her sergeant, who had been a deputy when she witnessed Nelly's jump, spoke with Nelly directly. She assured everyone that she had no intention of jumping again.

When I saw Nelly at pill call, she asked, "Do you remember me?"

"I do remember you. How are you doing?" I asked.

"My feet are quite painful, and I have arthritis, which also hurts," she replied.

She no longer had the drug-seeking urges she once did. She still relied on her orthopedic shoes to walk. Aging had not been kind to her, and she had developed several chronic illnesses over time.

I often wondered about inmates like Nelly, who seemed to know all the nursing staff and appeared happy to see us again upon their return to jail. Nelly seemed resigned to her circumstances, ready to serve her time without incident. Destiny in jail is unpredictable and brutally unequal—some survive, and others, despite support, do not.

> ***Life is like a box of chocolates.***
> ***You never know what you're going to get.***
> -Forest Gump

A Man to a Zombie in 45 Minutes

Minh took his weekly nine-pill TB dose without complaint. Minutes later, he returned flushed, trembling, and in pain. He said it happened every week. I called the doctor immediately; the medication was stopped, and follow-up was arranged. His quiet endurance was humbling—and a reminder of how easily serious reactions can be overlooked.

Let me tell you about another wild night at Oakwood – this time from the men's side of things. You know how some stories just stick with you? Well, this is definitely one of those.

It was a typical evening in men's medium-security lockdown, consisting of about 60 inmates in each of the four dorms, and I was busy with my normal nursing routine. I started the evening with pill call, as usual.

Minh, a tall, thin Vietnamese man, was in line to take his TB meds. The medical protocols had recently changed. Instead of giving TB meds twice a week with four pills each time (of Isoniazid and Pyridoxine), we were now doing a once-a-week dose with 9 tablets, a mix of Rifampin, Isoniazid, and Pyridoxine. Minh swallowed his weekly nine-pill TB dose with the quiet fortitude of someone used to suffering. I had no clue what was about to unfold.

I completed pill call and proceeded with my assessments – blood pressure checks, dressing wounds, and monitoring patients detoxing from alcohol to make sure they were detoxing safely. Just another typical evening, so I thought. I finished documentation in the medical office.

I barely had time to chart before deputies rushed him back, transformed into a flushed, trembling, pain-stricken version of himself, barely able to function. He looked like a creature pulled from a zombie film—eyes bloodshot, joints stiff, voice thin with agony. Holy moly, was he a sight!

This was NOT the same guy who had taken medications 45 minutes earlier. He complained of a sudden headache and joint pain. I checked his medical record; no known drug allergies were listed.

But here's where it gets really interesting. Minh looks at me and says, "Nurse, this happens to me every week! Just like this!" I was stunned. In 12 years of administering TB medications, I'd never seen anything like this. My heart broke. How many times had he cried alone behind steel doors because no one listened fully to his symptoms?

I took a moment to figure out which Standardized Procedure template to use to navigate this incident. There was no template. There *is* a procedure for administering TB medication, but this was totally different. This was a first for me. In my years working at Oakwood, I had given buckets of TB meds at pill call and had never seen a reaction to the medication.

Minh explained that he didn't react the first time, but since the second dose, he'd been experiencing these exact symptoms every single week, one to two hours after the dose. Tonight was the fastest reaction yet – just 45 minutes after taking the medication. He looked miserable. Minh had been taking these medications once a week for the last four weeks. Using his limited English, he quietly admitted he didn't want to continue taking the meds.

I checked his vital signs and immediately called the on-call MD. Healing shouldn't require such silent dedication. After hearing the details, the doctor gave a telephone order to discontinue the medications and scheduled an urgent appointment with the TB physician's assistant that same week.

I was still working in the medical office on the unit, cleaning up and checking the crash cart. One of the deputies called out, "Nurse, an inmate is having a seizure!" I left the office and was escorted into the dorm to see this inmate. The deputy who called me said, "It's the guy who reacted to the medicine you saw!" As I approached the bunk, I saw Minh curled up under a thin wool blanket, practically bouncing off the bunk with chills. I tried to speak to him. "Does this happen every week, too?" I asked.

Minh quietly responded, "Every week. It lasts five-six hours. Every week."

The deputies found a wheelchair, and Minh was rushed to Oakwood Medical for observation. There he began vomiting. A LOT! I asked, "Minh, every week?" He quietly replied, "Every week."

Digging through his medical records, I found previous documentation from nurses who had witnessed similar symptoms. The week before, they had merely noted "chills" and given him an appointment. The physician assistant had only slightly decreased one medication, not fully believing it was a severe reaction.

A few days later, I saw the on-call MD who had handled Minh's case that night. He was shocked, speculating that Minh was extremely sensitive to the medication; he couldn't believe he had been taking it for weeks with such intense symptoms.

My heart broke for Minh. Here was a patient suffering week after week, enduring these terrible reactions, and somehow managing to communicate his experience with such quiet persistence. I felt terrible that he had been going through this for so long. His quiet endurance humbled me; it also showed how easily dangerous reactions can be overlooked in a busy system.

I never got to follow up and see how he was doing, but I knew this was a patient I wouldn't forget anytime soon. His story was a powerful reminder that sometimes, medical experiences can be complex, personal, and far more intense than they might appear on the surface. In the world of healthcare, especially in settings like Oakwood, every patient has a story. Sometimes, those stories are more profound and challenging, and more human, than we might initially recognize.

> ***We know what we are,***
> ***but not what we may be.***
> -William Shakespeare

Bright Green Foam Everywhere

"Man down with green foam from his mouth." We ran and found him convulsing, neon foam bubbling from his lips. He swallowed cleaning solution after a phone call. We stabilized him and sent him to the ER. He survived — but the image haunted me long after.

"Man down! Inmate is on the ground with green foam oozing out of his mouth and nose. Awake and breathing. Code 3 called. Need medical response immediately," yelled a terrified voice over the radio.

I had finished my assignment, which included pill call, assessments, and an occasional inmate who came to the nurse with an upper respiratory infection or a toothache. But I was still at Oakwood Medical to help out if anyone needed assistance.

The nurses at Medical were trying to comprehend the meaning of the words we'd heard. We had a terrible feeling about what might be happening. Another nurse and I jumped into the electric car and rushed to the dorm. The deputies held the doors open for us to save time.

The two of us who had just arrived went to the building medical office, got the crash cart, and sprinted to the dorm. The assigned nurse was with the patient. The look in both their eyes was disturbing.

What we found was inconceivable: a man in his 40s, lying on the ground with a large volume of fluorescent green foam bubbling out of his mouth and nose!

A complete look of terror in his eyes.

The assigned nurse worked feverishly to clear the frothy foam to establish a clear airway. We got the patient's vital signs and started an IV in his arm.

The deputies reported that the patient had gotten “bad news” on the phone earlier that night and went into the bathroom, found a bottle of cleaning solution, and proceeded to ingest the contents of the bottle in a suicide attempt. The deputies gave us the bottle of fluid. Oakwood has to be careful in its choices of cleaners, for this precise reason!

I ran to the computer and printed out the Safety Data Sheet for the ER staff. Safety Data Sheets are required for substances used in the workplace and include first aid instructions, composition/ingredients, exposure controls/personal protection, measures of toxicity, and other considerations needed during an untoward event involving a hazardous compound. This allows the ER staff to facilitate treatment when they understand the exact nature of the chemicals ingested.

Another round of horrified faces ensued when the nurse briefed emergency personnel. The paramedics quickly followed with the gurney to transport the patient to the ER. This was a significant medical emergency. The patient was taken to my beloved Medical Center Level 1 Trauma Center.

The nurses began to clean up the area of medical supplies. The deputies investigated how the bottle of cleaner had ended up in the bathroom area. As we restocked the crash cart and medical office supplies, we were still shell-shocked to have experienced this very traumatic event.

As I shared, this devastated man had gotten some “bad news” over the phone; we didn’t know the details. We notified Mental Health to include them in the process. And we shared the information when we got back to Medical. The incident had initially been deemed a medical emergency, but it was a full-on suicide attempt. It was overwhelming.

The nurses found out that the patient received a tracheotomy and required several surgeries to repair the damage done by the fluid. He eventually came back to his dorm two months later.

I rotated assignments to that building during my years as a nurse at Oakwood. Every time I ended up at the dorm where this happened,

I could still see the man on the floor with all the bright green foam and the look of terror in his eyes. Those who responded to this incident saw things we couldn't unsee. I made several trips to the MH office to speak with coworkers and therapists who helped me deal with the trauma. I eventually got to the point where the image no longer haunted me.

This story reminds me of a patient I had as a nurse's aide in the 1970s at my beloved Medical Center. Trudy, a woman in her early 20s, was admitted after she attempted suicide by ingesting a corrosive liquid drain cleaner. The MDs worked feverishly to save her life. Many weeks after her admission, she was transferred out to our post-operative floor from the Intensive Care Unit. She wasn't able to eat and was given intravenous fluids. She was close to my age, and I couldn't imagine trying to commit suicide only to survive and have to experience the pain of this kind of trauma.

The MDs had done their best to clean out the necrotic tissue caused by the corrosive material. Still, hydrochloric gastric acid from her stomach leaked through her abdominal incision, causing painful irritation to the surrounding skin. The MDs devised the idea of applying baby food to the incision so the gastric acid would ingest it instead of the skin. So I watched the RNs smear baby food paste on her incision every day. The skin started to improve after a few days. Trudy suffered a lot. We all got to know her as she was in our care for weeks before her eventual discharge.

I was very impressed by the MDs' innovative solution. I hope Trudy got some help for whatever put her in the hospital in the first place.

Make a determination
that you will live your purpose today.
-Daniel Budzinski

Janie

She was heartbreak in human form — young, bipolar, and adrift. One day, she banged her head until she saw "black spots," sending me into a rapid neuro check. Another time, she swallowed a powdered cleanser like a confused child. Each encounter left me wondering what adulthood would look like since her life was already this chaotic.

Janie was an inmate in her twenties who had been arrested many times, so the Oakwood Medical and Mental Health departments knew her well. She was diagnosed with unspecified Bipolar Disorder and had trouble getting along with other inmates, so she was housed in a single cell. Young, bipolar, and lost in a world she didn't understand. When she got "program" time outside her cell, it was always by herself. Her only interactions were with the custody, medical, and mental health staff. Honestly, she seemed to prefer being alone, and she kept herself entertained.

If Janie complained of feeling suicidal, the deputies notified Mental Health. But when Janie physically hurt herself, they called Medical first.

One day, I was called to check on Janie after she repeatedly hit her head against the wall. She told us she was seeing black spots. The deputies warned her to stop, even threatening to call in the ERT (Emergency Response Team) to make her stop. Janie didn't listen. When the ERT arrived, she was shackled and moved to a safe spot where she couldn't keep hurting herself.

My job was to assess her injuries. She had minor scrapes on her forehead. Her pupils reacted equally to light, which indicated no neurological impairment. She was fully oriented; she knew the time, and who and where she was. Her hand grip and leg strength were strong and equal on both sides. But Janie complained of a slight headache and kept seeing those black spots. I notified the on-call MD, who was familiar with Janie's history. There were no new orders other than to monitor her for two hours and report any changes.

Janie sat quietly in waist chains, alone in a room with observation windows. Two hours later, Janie was returned to her cell.

Later that same night, a deputy let her spend about 15 minutes alone outside on the patio for some fresh air. A couple of hours after that, another deputy called to report that Janie was vomiting. I responded to her cell. She admitted to having tasted some powdered cleanser, like a confused child. She'd found it near a sink while she was on the patio. The powder was used for cleaning and ant control.

Janie had taken two small tastes and started feeling sick a couple of hours later. I checked her vitals—they were normal. Her vomit was just clear, foamy liquid in her toilet. I asked, "Have you eaten anything else that might've caused the vomiting?" "No," she said.

I grabbed the cleanser container and called Poison Control. I told them what Janie had said and gave them the product details so they could check the ingredients. Turns out, the cleanser was similar to a powdered antacid, so tasting it shouldn't have caused her to vomit. Still, because her vomiting wouldn't stop, Poison Control suggested sending her to the ER.

During my five-minute phone call, I could still hear Janie vomiting. I updated the on-call doctor. He approved sending her to the ER. I made the transport arrangements and informed Mental Health that she'd ingested the powder. Poison Control had confirmed it wasn't toxic, but it was up to Mental Health to decide whether this was a suicide attempt. If it were, Janie might need to be transferred to the Acute Psych Unit for evaluation.

I didn't follow up on what happened next—I was busy writing up my two encounters with Janie from that shift. A nurse called from the ER to confirm that the ingestion wasn't the issue, but the persistent vomiting. I confirmed the patient had been sent for vomiting. The ER nurse indicated she was very friendly and not vomiting when she arrived.

There was another incident with Janie in which I wasn't directly involved. She decided to poop in a bucket instead of the toilet. That was more of a Hazmat situation than either Medical or Mental Health.

Sadly, Janie's behaviors didn't seem to improve while in jail. She was receiving medication that she willingly took every day. I couldn't help but wonder what her future would be like since her life was already this chaotic in her twenties.

> ***Live as if you were to die tomorrow.***
> ***Learn as if you were to live forever.***
> - Mahatma Gandhi

Caller With a History

A man known for threats repeatedly called while his mentally ill wife was in custody. He raged and demanded answers. My pulse quickened with every ring. Deputies walked me to my car that night. Sometimes the storm outside the walls is as unsettling as the one inside. It reminded me that instability isn't limited to inmates—families carry their own trauma.

One evening shift, as I sat at the front desk in my role as Charge Nurse, the phone rang. More than a decade into my career at Oakwood Medical, I had answered thousands of calls. But this one was unlike any other call I had ever gotten at work.

Even now, as I sit here typing, I feel the return of those all-too-familiar sensations that came with working in a jail setting: the tightening knot in my stomach, the uptick in heart rate, shallow breathing, the dry mouth. Though I've been retired for some time, recounting these stories has a way of summoning those memories, emotions, and sensations. The silver lining is knowing that the physical tension tends to subside by the end of each writing session.

That evening, the caller identified himself as the husband of one of our patients, a profoundly mentally ill woman well known to both Oakwood Medical and the Mental Health departments. His voice was laced with anger and threats. He insisted he needed to speak with someone from the Probation Department. Given how busy the phones were, I transferred him to our supervisor. But he quickly called back, stating he refused to leave messages because "no one ever calls me back."

My coworker and I attempted to explain that Oakwood Medical was not affiliated with the Probation Department. Undeterred, he called back *TEN MORE TIMES*, each conversation showing up more agitated than the last. Eventually, we transferred his call to the Medical Deputy, who explained that his repeated harassing calls could lead to legal consequences. After that, the calls finally stopped, for the time being.

We were no strangers to this man. He had a long history of contacting various county departments, often threatening violence to anyone he was speaking to, and the staff in general. His name was so notorious that a memo had been circulated at both Oakwood Medical and Mental Health. Staff were instructed not to engage with him and to report any communication directly to Internal Affairs. IA was actively documenting every instance of his harassment of each county office.

Later that evening, the Medical Deputy asked if we would consider filing a formal complaint against the caller. We declined, noting that while his tone had been hostile and unrelenting, he hadn't explicitly threatened us with violence.

Still, our concern lingered. That night, as we prepared to leave work, we were uneasy about walking to our cars in the dark, public parking lot. We requested an escort from the deputies, who readily agreed. Thanks to their support, we left without incident—but the experience left an impression that never quite fades. It reminded me that instability isn't limited to inmates—families carry their own trauma.

> ***Never let one bad apple make you feel like everyone's gonna be bananas.***

Who Called 9-1-1?

A full fire response descended on Oakwood after an inmate secretly dialed 911 from a payphone, convinced it was the only way to be heard. Deputies warned him that misusing 911 can bring charges and endanger others. Beneath the poor choice, I saw something else — desperation disguised as defiance.

It was just another quiet evening at Oakwood. Until it wasn't.

The radio crackled at the East Gate. Deputy Carlson, leaning back in his chair with a lukewarm cup of coffee, straightened as he heard the unmistakable tone of urgency in Dispatch's voice.

"East Gate, be advised. Fire Department en route to your location, Code 3. ETA three minutes."

East Gate is the entry for deputies transporting inmates, trucks with mail, commissary supplies, meals for inmates, office supplies, deputies from other counties coming to pick up and transfer inmates to another facility, and other official vehicles, including emergency response.

Carlson blinked and sat upright. "Fire Department?" he said aloud, glancing out the gatehouse window. Sure enough, red lights were already visible at the far end of the road. He grabbed his radio.

"Control, this is East Gate," Carlson said. "I've got Engine 12 inbound Code 3. What's the emergency?"

There was a brief pause. The Control deputy was obviously confused.

"Stand by," Control replied. A few seconds passed. "We didn't call them. Checking with Medical..."

Carlson stared at the firetruck barreling toward the gate. "Well, someone sure did," he muttered.

A minute later, Control came back on the radio. "East Gate, Fire says they received a 911 call. Originated from a pay phone; location pings from Lockdown."

"That's an inmate building!" Carlson said, incredulous. "You're telling me an inmate called 9-1-1?"

"That's what they're saying," Control confirmed. "Medical's rolling to the dorm now. See if the deputies inside can identify who made the call."

Carlson buzzed the gate open just in time for the fire truck to roll through, sirens fading as it approached the inner gate. He shook his head. "This is gonna be a mess."

Inside Lockdown, Deputies Ramirez and Lacey were already moving.

"Who called 9-1-1?" Ramirez asked, raising his voice as he stepped into the common area. Several inmates looked up, startled. "Let's make this easy."

From the corner of the room, one of the inmates, a young man with glasses and a scowl, stood up slowly.

"I did," he said, arms crossed.

Ramirez narrowed his eyes. "You did? Why?"

"Because I've been telling the nurses for *days* something's wrong," the inmate snapped. "They didn't listen. My stomach hurts, I can't sleep, and nobody's doing a damn thing. So, I figured if no one around here cares, maybe 911 would."

Lacey glanced at Ramirez. "You've got to be kidding me."

Ramirez keyed his mic. "Control, be advised, we've got the caller ID'd. Inmate says he called 911 because Medical didn't take his complaints seriously."

Control replied, "Copy. Fire is en route to the dorm now. Medical's already on scene."

Within moments, the nurses arrived with their equipment. One of them, Nurse Tom, stepped up to the inmate.

"Let's take a look at you," he said briskly. "Sit down."

He conducted a full assessment while the fire crew stood by with their gear, exchanging skeptical looks.

After several minutes, Tom stood and addressed the deputies. "Vitals are stable. No acute distress. He doesn't need transport."

The fireman sighed. "Copy that. We'll clear out."

As the crew packed up, Deputy Ramirez turned to the inmate.

"You realize this isn't how things work, right?"

"I was desperate," the inmate said, shoulders tense. "Nobody listens."

"There's a chain of command," Ramirez said. "This stunt just pulled emergency services off the street. People could've died while they were dealing with *this*."

The inmate looked away, saying nothing.

The usual sequence of events, when calling for the Fire Department, is that the deputy calls for Medical to respond. If it's obvious to the deputy that this is an emergency, the deputy will notify Control right before calling Medical. Nurses respond to the patient. Control calls 911.

Within just a few minutes, Control notifies 911 of the nature and location of the emergency. They inform the East Gate deputy of the impending emergency response, including the location, so they can give directions when Fire/ambulance arrive. Control then opens gates to the emergency location. Control also assigns a deputy to accompany the patient if transport to the ER is necessary.

Later, back at the gate, Carlson relayed the whole event to another deputy coming on shift.

“So let me get this straight,” the deputy said, raising an eyebrow. “An inmate didn’t like the nurses’ response...and just dialed 911?”

Carlson nodded. “That’s the short version.”

“What happens to him now?”

Carlson shrugged. “No idea. But I wouldn’t be surprised if charges are filed.”

He took a sip of his now-cold coffee and muttered, “Next time he complains about stomach pain, it might just be from stress. Because that little call? Gonna cause a whole lot of paperwork.”

> ***The first 5 days after the weekend are always the hardest.***
>
> -Jimmy Buffett

How to Touch Up Grey Hair Behind Bars

She grinned like she'd found buried treasure. "Look," she whispered, running a hand through her newly tinted hair, "instant coffee and grape Kool-Aid." The reddish-brown actually suited her. Her pride over that small victory reminded me how fiercely people crave autonomy when every choice is stripped away. Beauty isn't frivolous — it's survival.

It was late afternoon in the women's dorm, just before dinner. I was setting up for diabetic call, pulling out the glucometer and alcohol swabs, as the usual line of women began to form. Most of them knew the routine—line up, finger prick, quick number check, and off to meds or dinner. We saw each other almost every day during blood sugar testing and pill call, so I'd gotten to know them—at least a little.

That's probably why I noticed one of the middle-aged ladies right away.

As she stepped up, something about her looked different. Same khaki uniform, same calm expression—but something had changed.

"You look different today," I said, squinting slightly, trying to figure it out.

She smiled, pleased. "You noticed!"

I tilted my head. "Did you—did you do something to your hair?"

She nodded, her smile growing wider. "Sure did. Covered up the grays."

I blinked. "Wait, you dyed your hair? In here?"

"Yep," she said, clearly proud of herself. "Used a little jailhouse chemistry."

I chuckled. "Now you've got me curious."

She leaned in slightly and lowered her voice, like she was sharing a family secret: "Instant coffee and grape Kool-Aid."

I raised an eyebrow. "Seriously?"

"Dead serious," she replied. "Mixed it up into a paste, slathered it on, let it sit about half an hour, then washed it out."

"And it works?" I asked, still a bit stunned.

She tilted her head with a small shrug. "Better than nothing. Covered the grays. Gave me a nice kind of reddish-brown tint. Smells like breakfast, though."

We both laughed.

I glanced down at the glucometer. "Well, I have to say, it looks good. You did a great job."

"Thanks," she said. "You've got to get creative in here. We don't have much, but we make it work."

Her words stuck with me. They often did.

Later, after diabetic call was complete and I was tidying up, I kept thinking about her. The makeshift hair dye was more than just a clever trick—it was a quiet act of defiance, a way to hold onto a sense of identity in a place designed to strip it away. A little color to tint a gloomy gray world.

In the free world, we have endless options. In here, they have ingenuity.

> ***Do not take life too seriously.***
> ***You will never get out of it alive.***
> - Elbert Hubbard

That's Not a Handball

During a handball game, something skidded across the yard — a breast implant. A transgender inmate had collided mid-game, and the implant ruptured free. Custody logged it as a "Patient-Owned Silicone Prosthetic" and sent her to the ER. Even now, I shake my head at the surrealness of that shift.

The day started like most others—or at least as what passes for normal around here. At 3 p.m., I checked in for the swing shift and headed straight to the med room. Diabetic Call always came first, and we had our usual crowd—some chatty, some cranky, all impatient.

I was halfway through testing when the radio crackled to life.

"Control to Medical, man down—Protective Custody dorm, Lockdown Yard. Medical response requested immediately."

I paused with a lancet in hand. I looked up, instinctively alert.

"We got it," came the reply from one of the RNs already on the scene.

The tension in the room dipped slightly. "Guess it's handled," I said, turning back to my next patient.

But nothing is ever just "handled" at Oakwood. Not really.

Later, during dinner break, I sat in the staff lounge with my reheated leftovers when Nurse Jackie dropped into the seat across from me, eyes wide and laughing silently.

"You're not gonna believe what that 'man down' call was about..."

"Try me," I said. I was eating soft foods, recovering from an orthodontic appointment, so I was stirring my mashed potatoes with more interest than usual.

"Okay, so Protective Custody had a handball game going. One of the inmates—you know, Miranda? Middle-aged, short, red bangs, always carrying that tattered romance novel?"

I nodded. "Yeah, the one going through gender reassignment?"

"That's her. Still legally listed as male, but presenting female. So, apparently, she's in the game, full energy, when she crashes into a couple of guys mid-play. Big collision."

"Oof."

"Yeah, except when she hit the ground, one of her breast implants *literally* popped out of her chest."

"Wait—what?!"

"I'm serious! It launched like a rogue dodgeball. Hit the concrete and rolled toward the fence."

I nearly choked on a mouthful of green beans.

"You're making this up."

"I swear on my nursing license. The other guys didn't know what to do. One of them yelled, 'Yo! What the hell is that?!' and someone else said, 'That ain't no handball!'"

We both burst out laughing, but quickly muffled ourselves. This place had ears everywhere.

"So what happened next?"

"Well, Miranda was clutching her chest, bleeding through her jumpsuit. Med team rolled in fast. She was calm, though, just said, 'I think I lost something important.'"

"Oh my god," I muttered.

"They took her to the ER to get the wound cleaned and sutured. The implant was intact, somehow. We had to log it into her property as a personal item."

"Do you...do you just write 'breast implant' on the inventory sheet?"

"Nope. Officially labeled as: 'Silicone Prosthetic, Patient-Owned, Left Side.'" She smirked. "Admin wanted to know if we should refrigerate it."

"Stop it."

"I'm not kidding. One of the officers asked if it could be used as contraband—like, weaponized. I told him only if she slings it in a sock."

We sat in silence for a second before dissolving into giggles again.

Welcome to Oakwood. Where no day is typical, and sometimes, the strangest part of your shift is filling out a form for a breast implant that tried to play handball. Even now, I can't think about that day without shaking my head in disbelief.

Keep situations, thoughts, and feelings in perspective. Wait for things to unravel before you act.

- Betterhelp.com

My Mattress Is Too Thin

Inmates often complained about their thin mattresses, but one woman got creative. She hoarded fiber packets and stuffed them under her mattress for padding. After that, we had to open every packet we dispensed. I couldn't even be angry. When your world is cement and steel, comfort is precious. Ingenuity fills the gaps.

Mattresses in jails are intended for repeated use. They are characteristically thin and covered with thick plastic. They are routinely cleaned after each inmate's use. Inmates frequently complain about difficulty sleeping due to their assigned bedding's lack of comfort and support.

“Man, I can't get any sleep on this thing,” one inmate muttered during morning rounds, rubbing his back. “It's like sleeping on a slab of ice.”

Oakwood nurses conduct daily assessments to monitor and address inmate health, including illness, injury, mental health, medical, and dental concerns. Nurses are expected to memorize and apply procedures for managing the most common inmate complaints.

“Let me guess,” Nurse Karen said with a tired smile during her morning shift, clipboard in hand, “constipation again?”

One prevalent complaint is indeed constipation. When an inmate reports this issue, nurses carry out a complete assessment to eliminate more serious medical conditions. If no contraindications are found, the standard response is to start a fiber regimen, where the inmate receives a package containing a dose of powdered fiber supplement twice daily for 14 days.

“We’ll start you on fiber,” she explained, handing a cup to an inmate. “You mix it with water, like this. Drink it all, twice a day.”

The proper administration method for the fiber supplement is for the nurse to empty the contents of the packet into a cup and instruct the inmate to mix it with water. However, over time, this practice deteriorated. Nurses began distributing the unopened packets directly to inmates instead of preparing the doses as instructed. Most inmates did as they were told.

But one afternoon, when deputies were performing a routine “shakedown,” they lifted up a mattress to look for contraband.

“What the hell?” one deputy exclaimed, holding up a layer of colorful fiber packets stashed beneath it. “Why are these under your bed?”

The inmate, a young woman with a weary face, shrugged. “It’s too uncomfortable,” she replied. “I used it for padding so I could sleep better.”

This misuse led to disciplinary action against the inmate and the confiscation of the contraband fiber. The event also prompted the facility to reinforce proper dispensing protocols.

“Effective immediately,” the nurse manager announced during the staff meeting, “all fiber packets must be opened and emptied into a cup before being handed to an inmate. No exceptions.” A reminder was circulated to all nursing staff, emphasizing the policy to ensure both compliance and the intended therapeutic effect.

> ***It amazes me how much exercise and extra fries sound alike.***
>
> \- Anonymous

Fashion Behind Bars

A clothing mix-up sent oversized garments into maximum security, and the women turned the dorm into a runway. Laughter bounced off concrete as shirts became gowns and "jailhouse capris." For a moment, the weight of incarceration lifted, replaced by creativity and joy — glimpses of who these women were beyond the walls.

I had been working as a nurse at Oakwood Correctional Facility for several years before I noticed the subtle rhythms of inmate life, the small rituals that gave structure to their days. One such routine was clothing exchange day. Every week, inmates submitted requests for clean clothes, specifying their sizes. In return, deputies collected the worn garments and issued replacements. The system worked well enough. Though like anything involving paper forms and human hands, it wasn't without the occasional mistake.

One Monday afternoon, a mix-up found its way to the max security women's dormitory. These were long-term residents, most of them waiting years as their serious charges wound their way through the courts. By now, they knew each other well. Jokes were shared like cigarettes, and humor was one of the few currencies no one could confiscate.

That day, someone had received a 5X T-shirt—far too large for any of the women on that tier.

"Who ordered a tent?" a voice called out as one of the deputies handed the bundle through the gate.

Laughter rippled across the dorm. A woman named Tamika held up the massive shirt, letting it billow out in front of her.

“Dang, y’all! I think I just got me a new wardrobe!” she said, grinning.

Tamika wasn’t one to let an opportunity pass. She slipped her arms through the sleeves, then twisted the neck of the shirt behind her head like a halter strap. With a dramatic twirl, she strutted down the narrow aisle between bunks, the shirt sweeping the floor like the train of a ballgown.

“Look at her, look at her!” someone shouted.

“You better work it, Miss Beverly Hills!” another inmate called, clapping her hands.

Tamika lifted her chin and placed one hand delicately on her hip. “This? Oh, just something I picked up on Rodeo Drive,” she said with mock elegance. “Very exclusive. Cotton-poly blend, darling.”

For a few minutes, the entire dorm roared with laughter. It wasn’t just funny, it was liberating. The gray walls seemed less oppressive, the uniforms less identical. In that moment, Tamika wasn’t Inmate #44782. She was a woman in her mansion, gliding across marble floors in her designer dressing gown.

A few days later, another oversized tee found its way to the same dorm. This time it was Sierra, quiet and wiry, with a streak of cleverness behind her shy smile. She didn’t make a big show of it. She just stepped out of the bathroom one morning wearing the shirt in a completely new way.

“What in the world…?” someone muttered, doing a double-take.

Sierra had threaded her legs through the sleeves, pulled the body of the shirt up over her hips, and tied the hem around her waist. The result looked something like baggy lounge shorts.

Tamika, peering through the bars during the morning med line, cracked up. “Girl, those are *fire*! You just invented jailhouse capris!”

Sierra shrugged, but she was smiling. “Hey, it’s more comfortable than them state-issue drawers.”

For a few moments, Sierra walked a little taller. Heads turned. Compliments were whispered. In a place where sameness was mandatory and individuality suppressed, looking "different"—even if only for a minute—was revolutionary.

Later, I found myself thinking about those two women and their makeshift outfits. The clothes weren't special, but what they made of them was. It was fashion, yes, but more than that, it was resistance. It was imagination. And it was proof that even behind bars, creativity doesn't get locked down.

> ***Fashion is what you buy.***
> ***Style is what you do with it***
> - Quotes.com

Crocheting in Jail

When Lana proposed crocheting NICU blankets, hope entered the dorm. Women gathered with yarn at their feet, stitching and sharing stories. "Stitches of Hope" gave them purpose. In a place that strips identity, it helped them reclaim a piece of it.

Several years ago, an amazing woman named Lana was transferred from prison to Oakwood, hoping to appeal her conviction. She was placed in the max security housing unit. There was a calm confidence about her that stood out. She walked into the unit with purpose, like she carried something more than just her legal burdens. She carried hope.

One afternoon, I overheard her speaking to Sergeant Miller near the unit entrance.

"Sergeant," Lana said, her voice steady but gentle, "I wanted to ask if I could share an idea with you. It's something we did in prison that really helped keep us focused and out of trouble—and it made a big difference."

Sergeant Miller raised an eyebrow. "I'm listening."

"There was a program," Lana continued, "where inmates who had good behavior and could be trusted were given crochet hooks and yarn. We made blankets for children in hospitals—for kids with cancer, and babies in the NICU. It gave us purpose. We weren't just waiting for time to pass. We were doing something that mattered."

Sergeant Miller crossed her arms but didn't look away. "Crochet hooks, huh? That's...different."

"I know it sounds unusual," Lana said with a smile. "But you'd be surprised how seriously the women take it. It gave them a reason to stay out of trouble. Some of us hadn't felt useful in years—until that yarn passed through our fingers."

The sergeant was quiet for a moment, then gave a short nod. "All right. I'll run it up the chain. We'll need to figure out the logistics—who can be trusted, how to get supplies. But it's worth looking into."

Within weeks, the unit was buzzing. Word spread quickly that Lana's idea had been approved, and a list was quietly passed around for women to sign up. The staff worked with community partners to gather donated yarn. A local church group agreed to help. Hooks and patterns were collected. I hadn't heard any of this officially, but I began to notice more and more women sitting together, their hands working carefully, colorful yarn winding between their fingers.

It wasn't until I ran into Sergeant Miller during an afternoon diabetic call that I found out what was going on.

"I see all the crocheting happening," I said casually. "What's the story?"

The sergeant grinned. "Lana's idea took off. They're making baby blankets for the NICU at your Medical Center. Can you believe it?"

I gasped. "That's *my* hospital. Oh, those little babies...They need warmth. Comfort. That's incredible."

"Yeah," she said. "We're calling it *Stitches of Hope.* And let me tell you—they love it. You should see their faces."

"Can I donate yarn or hooks?" I asked quickly, already thinking through which craft stores I could hit that weekend.

Sergeant Miller's answer came fast, a resounding "Yes. Please."

So, I went shopping like a woman on a mission. I bought every pastel shade I could find—soft blues, buttery yellows, lilacs, mint greens. I scooped up crochet hooks in every size. When I dropped everything off with the sergeant, she looked at the haul and laughed.

"You weren't kidding."

"These babies deserve softness," I said, tearing up. "And the women deserve to know they're still capable of doing something good."

Weeks went by, and every time I stepped into the max security dorm—whether during diabetic call or night pill line—I saw the transformation happening. Women who had once sat staring at the walls or anxiously pacing now gathered together in quiet clusters. They chatted, encouraged each other, and held up their work with pride.

One evening, I sat down next to a woman named Tasha, who was crocheting a lavender and white blanket. "That's beautiful," I said.

"Thanks," she replied, not looking up. "I've never done anything like this before."

"Were you nervous to start?"

She gave a short laugh. "Terrified. I thought I'd mess it up. But Lana showed me. And now I can't stop."

"Do you know where that blanket's going?"

"To a baby in the hospital," she said softly. "A tiny one who needs help staying warm."

She paused, then added, "I never thought I'd be the one giving comfort to someone else. Not in here." That stuck with me.

After each blanket was finished, Sergeant Miller would take a picture of the maker holding it up proudly. She created a large display on a bulletin board in the main hall—a collage of women and their creations, surrounded by cut-out hearts and stars. Anyone passing by could see the joy in their eyes.

Some blankets were vibrant and creative, others more modest and simple—but each was full of care. Full of love. *Stitches of Hope* became a sanctuary. Women who rarely spoke began confiding in one another. The women learned, created, shared stories, and found purpose. Watching their pride grow was deeply moving. Their hands worked gently, lovingly, weaving purpose into each thread. When we posted photos of them holding their finished blankets, pride glowed on their faces. In a place designed to strip people of identity, this program gave them a piece of themselves back.

I often stopped at that photo display, just to look. And each time, I felt that familiar lump in my throat. Lana's idea had done more than just fill idle hands—it had stitched a thread of purpose through a place often defined by waiting and regret.

"Lana," I said to her once, catching her in the hallway, "I hope you know how much this means. You changed something here."

She smiled, holding a half-finished pink blanket in her lap. "We all need to feel like we matter. Even in here." And thanks to her, they did.

> ***You must expect great things of yourself before you can do them***
>
> \- Michael Jordan

Special Requests for Housing

Re-housing requests usually came with fear, but sometimes with humor. Craig, a Type 1 diabetic, pleaded to stay in Lockdown rather than move to minimum — he couldn't handle the "smell and chaos of 60 men." Devin, afraid of mice, tried to give up his lower bunk because "mice stay on the floor." Beneath the jokes, I heard something deeper — men grasping for small pockets of comfort in a place that offered little.

The inmates at Oakwood arrive after they have been booked and processed. Some stay only a few days before posting bail. Others find themselves stuck in limbo—waiting for court dates, waiting for answers, waiting for something to change.

Craig had already been at Oakwood, housed in Lockdown for months, awaiting his sentencing. A Type 1 diabetic in his late twenties, he was tall, lean, and—by most accounts— handsome. His polite manner set him apart. Even in Lockdown, where tension simmered constantly just below the surface, Craig managed to be respectful and composed. Nurses saw him four times a day for his blood sugar checks.

"Morning, Craig," said Nurse Letty as she snapped on a pair of gloves. She liked him. He never gave her trouble.

"Hey, Nurse Letty. Blood sugar bingo, right?" he said, holding out his finger with a crooked grin.

"You know the drill."

He winced slightly as the lancet pricked his skin. "How's the outside world treating you?" he asked.

"About the same as in here, just with worse traffic," Letty replied.

Craig chuckled, but his eyes always had a watchful stillness—like he was seeing things a few layers deeper than most.

One morning, shortly after his sentencing, he stopped by Medical with a strange request.

"I heard I'm getting moved to Minimum," he said to the on-duty nurse, scratching the back of his neck awkwardly.

"That's standard for your level of custody," she said, flipping through the chart. "You'll be in the barracks."

"Yeah... about that." He shifted in his chair. "Can I stay in Lockdown instead?"

The nurse raised an eyebrow. "You want to *stay* in Lockdown?"

Craig nodded earnestly. "I know it sounds weird, but I was in Minimum for a couple nights before court. Those barracks—60 guys in one room—smelled like a chili cook-off gone wrong. The farting never stops."

There was a beat of silence. "You're serious?" the nurse said, suppressing a laugh.

"Completely. At least in Lockdown, there are only two guys to a cell. There's a door. And some air circulation."

The nurse sighed. "Well, it's not up to us. We'll submit the request, but Custody's probably going to laugh this one off."

And they did. The denial came back within a day: *Request denied. Inmate to be housed according to standard classification.*

***

A second inmate who was housed in the minimum barracks came to Medical one day with a housing change request. His name was Devin, a wiry guy in his early twenties with restless hands and anxious eyes. He had a heart condition. Because of his cardiac diagnosis, the Medical department was authorized to request that the inmate be housed in a valuable “lower bunk” housing. Lower bunks were preferred by many inmates for their accessibility.

“I need to talk to someone about my housing assignment,” he said in a low voice.

Nurse Letty opened his chart in the computer. “You’ve got medical clearance for a lower bunk due to your heart condition. What’s the issue?”

“I, uh...” He hesitated, clearly embarrassed. “I want to cancel my lower bunk assignment.”

Letty blinked. “You want to give up a *lower bunk*? People beg for those.”

“I know. I know. But I’ve seen, like, three mice this week. And they’re always on the floor. I swear one ran over my shoe last night.”

“Mice?”

“Yes! I’d rather sleep higher up where they don’t go.”

Letty looked at him, then at the chart. “Your heart condition doesn't care about mice.”

“I'll take my chances.”

She sighed and scribbled some notes. "I’ll send it in, but I can already tell you the answer."

Sure enough, Medical denied the change. Devin trudged back to the barracks. Ironically, his heart was pounding at the thought of little gray feet skittering beneath him in the dark.

Inmates had all kinds of reasons for wanting to be where they weren’t—some medical, some practical, and some purely human. But Oakwood, as ever, had rules. And the rules didn’t make room for flatulence or mice.

Dear Karma, I have a list of people you missed
- Author unknown

You Need to Put This Where?

A Lesson in Unexpected Care

A transgender woman had surgery prior to incarceration. The Gyn MD ordered daily vaginal dilation. The glass dilator had to be stored and supervised for security. I explained the sterile process; she nodded, reassuring me she'd done it before. The vulnerability between us was quiet but profound. Gender-affirming care in jail demands a tenderness no one teaches you.

I was early in my shift when I reviewed the medical files and saw a name I recognized. She had been with us for a few weeks now—a woman in her twenties who had been placed in Protective Custody due to her gender identity. She had completed gender-affirming surgery prior to her incarceration and was medically, visibly, and legally female.

Her appearance was striking. She was beautiful in a way that caught people off guard—long dark hair, clear skin, a calm and gentle demeanor. But what made her memorable was not just how she looked; it was how she carried herself with quiet grace in a place designed to crush it.

That morning, she had an off-site appointment with a gynecologist. When she returned, there was a note from the physician detailing post-operative care. My eyes paused on one line:

"Patient must use vaginal dilator daily to maintain depth and elasticity of neovagina."

A dilator. Of course. I should have thought of that. The surgery created a vaginoplasty, which maintained elasticity when the woman was having sex. This wasn't the case behind bars. The inmate was instructed to use a glass cylindrical object daily to maintain the integrity of the tissue.

I met with the charge nurse and the facility sergeant to review the implications. Because the dilator was made of solid glass and could theoretically be used as a weapon, custody had to be looped into the logistics of storing, supervising, and transporting the device.

Later that day, I gathered the items—a sterile dilator, lubricant, gloves—and headed toward the protective custody holding cell where she was temporarily housed for the appointment.

I knocked gently before entering.

She looked up from her cot, her eyes alert but calm. “Hi,” she said.

“Hi,” I replied, trying to keep my tone steady. “I have the supplies from your doctor’s visit today.”

She sat up, smoothing her jumpsuit over her knees. “Okay.”

I hesitated, holding the kit in my gloved hands. “So...this is the dilator and lubricant your GYN ordered for daily use,” I explained, offering it to her. “I need to...explain how to use it.”

She gave me a warm, patient smile. “It’s okay,” she said softly. “I’ve used one before. I know how it works.”

“Oh. That’s—great.” I exhaled a little too quickly. “Thank you. I didn’t know if you’d need help.”

Her tone was gentle, but confident: “No worries. I’m glad you’re kind about it. Not everyone is.”

I was momentarily silent. There was nothing to say that didn’t feel inadequate.

She glanced at the items in my hands. “They’re letting me keep it in my cell?”

“We’ll coordinate with custody. It has to be stored securely and signed out when you need it, just like any other medical device with potential...risks.” I paused. “But yes, you’ll have access to it daily.”

The dilator was secured on the nurse's medication cart for use only during the pill call, then returned to the nurse.

"Good," she said. "It's important."

I nodded. "I understand."

Before I turned to go, I added, "If anything changes—if you experience pain, bleeding, or anything unusual—please tell us. You don't have to manage that alone."

She looked at me, eyes steady. "Thank you. I won't."

As I stepped back into the hallway, I took a deep breath and leaned against the cool concrete wall. I hadn't expected this part of nursing school to catch up with me here—not the anatomy or the procedure, but the human complexity of it all.

We're trained to take blood pressure, to dress wounds, to administer medications. But no one teaches you how to navigate dignity, identity, and trauma in a jail cell. No one furnishes a manual for you on how to hand a woman a glass instrument and preserve not just her anatomy, but her autonomy. In that moment, I didn't feel embarrassed anymore. I felt honored.

This wasn't just a medical procedure. It was a reminder of what nursing is really about—meeting people where they are, seeing them as they are, and caring for them completely.

Even—especially—when it's unexpected.

Some mornings I wake up grouchy.
Other mornings, I just let him sleep.

- unknown

Harold

Harold was lost in alcohol withdrawal, barely oriented — yet scheduled for release that night. I couldn't let him walk out into danger. Sgt. Heartfield listened and approved a courtesy ER transfer. He left alive and protected. I knew we had altered the course of his story. Maybe even saved his life.

The Universe is at it again, pushing me to places I've never been and expecting me to deliver.

I recently experienced a whirlwind of events that brought both joy and challenges. First, my son married his sweetheart in a fairy-tale wedding near the beach in Half Moon Bay, California. It was an unforgettable day filled with love and celebration.

Next came a "touchy-feely, hippy-dippy" weekend for a conference focused on spirituality and healing in Denver, Colorado. My niece and I attended class all day and spent our lunch break looking for a cannabis store to grab some souvenirs. When my niece forgot her ID in her suitcase, I had to go into the store alone without my niece to "school" me. In the end, everyone had a great time.

After that serene and rejuvenating week off, I returned to work with a song in my heart and a spring in my step. I was assigned to men's lockdown, which consisted of four dorms housing inmates of all ages and backgrounds. Flipping through pages of my binder with the MARs (Medical Administration Records), which listed medications each inmate was receiving, I came across an ETOH (alcohol withdrawal) protocol for an inmate born in 1940.

Yikes! An elderly detoxing inmate in Lockdown? This concerned me.

The notes indicated that Harold, the inmate, had been booked 24 hours earlier. The assessments showed a score of 0, meaning he had no hand tremors, no difficulty eating, and was oriented to his surroundings. I could not shake the thought: *How can a 74-year-old man safely navigate life in a dorm full of seasoned criminals?*

At pill call, I asked the COs (custody officers) about Harold. They complained, "He can't even remember how to get back to his bunk!" They let out a collective moan and begged me to rehouse him to Main Jail, where he could receive individualized care.

After finishing pill call, I interviewed Harold. He was a delightful man with a reddish tint to his hair.

"Are you eating okay?" I asked. "I have no trouble eating," he assured me.

When I tested his orientation, I asked where he was. He looked around the medical room, thought for a moment, and replied, "There's a big room with lots of bunks in it." He couldn't identify that he was in jail. "What year is it?" I continued. "2012!" He replied confidently. It was 2015.

His answers confirmed my concerns, which started the algorithm in my head to start his transfer to Main Jail. "I'm going to transfer you to a quieter setting so you can get some rest," I told Harold. He was delighted. I quickly finished with the other inmates and completed the Med/Psych referral to transfer him to safer housing. I carried the form to Lockdown Control to fax it to Classification, which would speed up the process of finding a deputy to transfer him.

The CO asked to see the document and declared, "I just got a fax that he's been cited out. He is released tonight!" My brain froze. Harold was too disoriented to be released safely.

I immediately called Classification, who confirmed his release paperwork was already with Processing.

Determined to find a solution, I headed to Processing, located next door to Medical, to ask how they planned to ensure his safety. CO

Allen suggested I check with Mental Health to see if they had any ideas.

By now, it was 10 p.m., and the night shift would start in an hour. Mental Health staff checked the computer and found no history to justify a Mental Health hold. The MH woman mentioned they had bus tokens, but he did not seem safe enough to negotiate public transit. Processing had taxi vouchers, but even a taxi posed risks.

CO Allen shared a chilling story: a month earlier, another elderly inmate had been released. Two hours later, the California Highway Patrol reported he'd been struck and killed while walking on the freeway. He had Oakwood release papers in his pocket!

Realizing the gravity of the situation, I escalated to Sgt. Heartfield. She instructed me to submit a Mental Health referral. MH said he couldn't be held for EPS (Emergency Psych Services) because he had no Mental Health diagnosis.

Sgt. Heartfield spoke to me directly. "Send him Code 1 to VMC ER," she said. "They'll ensure he's released safely."

I felt an immediate sense of relief! Harold would be sent to the ER as a courtesy transfer.

Harold was brought to Processing, dressed out, and taken to the ER by a CO. I called ahead to notify the Charge nurse about his condition.

That night, I reflected on how a few simple questions had sparked a complex process to secure Harold's safety. I learned a lot from the experience and was profoundly grateful for Sgt. Heartfield's guidance. Harold was now in good hands.

Only in the darkness can you see the stars.
-Martin Luther King, Jr.

12 Shades of Purple

During wound care for a post-op breast augmentation, a male deputy accidentally walked past as the patient lifted her shirt. He froze, blushed, and retreated in mortified silence. She, meanwhile, admired herself as if she were on a runway. Awkward, absurd, human — only in jail do pride and embarrassment collide so perfectly.

That particular night, I was working with recently incarcerated medium security women who were worried about their cases. They tended to exhibit more drama than the other female inmates and were, therefore, unpredictable. I never knew what unusual incident might occur during my shift.

The medical area was a carefully designed space of functionality and limited privacy. Three interconnected rooms housed essential medical equipment – crash cart, critical medical supplies, medicine carts, computers, and examination tables. Exam tables, without stirrups, are used for any assessments that require the patient to lie flat: wound care, assessing bowel sounds, listening to fetal heart tones, administering enemas, etc. The layout reflected the careful balance between medical needs and institutional security protocols.

I had finished pill call and handed the deputy my list of inmates who needed assessments. I was making my way through the list when a young woman entered the Medical room. I checked her armband and looked up her medical record on the computer. She had been arrested the day before. She told the Booking nurse she had surgery that day, and needed wound care. The Booking nurse assessed the surgery on her breasts and initiated MD orders to start antibiotic ointment on the incisions and cover them with a dry dressing two times a day. Her primary concern was protecting her recent surgical investment, a deeply personal medical procedure now complicated by her incarceration.

The room in Medical had an area for wound care, but the inmate requested more privacy than just the skimpy privacy screen positioned in the doorway. I appreciated her need for privacy, understanding how exposed and vulnerable one might feel in such circumstances. The privacy screen seemed inadequate, so we moved to the middle room – a neutral space between the medical exam areas.

A male deputy remained stationed in the hallway, maintaining standard safety protocols. Deputies are usually female in women's inmate dorms. Not tonight, though.

The inmate removed her cover top, thermal shirt, and bra. I collected the supplies I would need for wound care around the nipples as well as dressings to apply, washed and dried my hands, and put sterile gloves on.

"How does it look, Nurse?" the inmate asked.

"It looks like brand new incisions with no evidence of infection at all," I replied.

"I just had surgery yesterday, and I'm worried about getting an infection in this place," the inmate said with an audible tone of concern in her voice.

"As long as the incision is kept clean and covered, it should heal without any problems. Your oral antibiotic will add another level of protection from infection," I responded in an attempt to put an end to her fears. My words were meant to provide comfort, to remind her that despite her current circumstances, her health and personal care remained a priority.

As I was finishing up applying antibiotic ointment to the incisions around her nipples, I heard some commotion behind me. The deputy, always kind and thoughtful around inmates, was "standing by" in the hallway to make sure the inmates waiting for care didn't cause any trouble. I soon realized he'd decided to glance into the room. My back was to him as I completed wound care, but he had a full view of the young woman, with her breasts completely exposed!

The sudden exposure seemed to overwhelm him completely. His sympathetic nervous system kicked into high gear, and his face turned 12 shades of purple. He muttered an apology and practically fled the room.

His immediate reaction after fleeing was to go directly to his sergeant to report what had just happened! He asked to be reassigned for the remainder of his shift – a response that spoke volumes about the complex dynamics of professional boundaries and personal discomfort. No administrative action was taken as a result of the incident.

The inmate's reaction was surprisingly casual. She commented that she was so proud of her surgical results that she wouldn't mind walking around topless. I gently reminded her about behavioral consequences that could result in infractions, adding extra time to her sentence.

Years later, this moment remained etched in my memory. It wasn't just about a medical procedure or a momentary professional awkwardness. It was about human dignity, vulnerability, and the delicate balance of maintaining professional boundaries while acknowledging individual humanity.

The deputy's mortified reaction, the inmate's complex emotional response, and my role as a healthcare professional trying to provide compassionate care – all of these elements wove together to create a moment that transcended the typical institutional narrative.

This singular experience – my only patient with one-day-old breast surgery – became a poignant reminder of the deeply personal stories that unfold within institutional walls. Each interaction, no matter how brief, can reveal profound aspects of human resilience, vulnerability, and the universal desire to maintain one's sense of self, even under the most challenging circumstances.

Every time I encountered that deputy afterward, a private, knowing smile would cross my face – a silent acknowledgment of a moment that reminded us both of the unpredictable, deeply human nature of our work.

> ***Life itself is the most wonderful fairy tale.***
> - Hans Christian Anderson

Conclusion

When I look back on my 16 years at Oakwood, I feel gratitude braided with grief and awe. I entered as a nurse and left changed — shaped by inmates who trusted me, deputies who protected me, and coworkers who carried me through impossible shifts. I witnessed horror and resilience, cruelty and deep compassion. Writing these stories has turned haunting memories into ones that honor the lives within them. Oakwood continues without me, but its echoes remain. And I am truly grateful.

At Oakwood, it never failed: I'd walk away from an encounter with a patient—sometimes shaken, sometimes laughing, sometimes both—and think, *People would never believe this if they weren't here. I should write it down.* But I didn't. Not for years.

When my kids were little and said or did something cute, I used to scribble their funny sayings on scraps of paper and tuck them away. Years later, I found those little pieces of paper, and they brought back the BEST memories.

I never did that with my jail stories—until one day, a voice in my head nagged: *Write them. People have no idea what you do there.*

Once I started, I couldn't stop. I tested my idea on everyone from my doctor to my dentist, family, and even my favorite grocery checker, and the reaction was unanimous: *"Yes—tell these stories."* They encouraged me to keep going.

And once I retired, the memories came rushing back. Some were hilarious. Some were heartbreaking. Some were so outrageous they'll stay locked in my private files forever—because if I published them, I might be the one ending up in court.

Writing forced me to relive everything. I could picture the cells, hear the keys jangling, remember the sharp mix of adrenaline and compassion that defined each day. The more I wrote, the more my head memories slid into my heart. These weren't just "work stories" anymore; they were evidence of a career I never expected to love, in a place most people never imagine can be rewarding.

The public usually hears about fights, escapes, riots, deaths, and failures. What they don't hear is that behind those walls are staff who show up every day, balancing toughness with humanity, and sometimes offering an inmate the first scrap of dignity they've had in years. I wanted to make sure someone told *that* side.

To the custody staff who kept me safe, to my coworkers who shared the burden and these amazing experiences—thank you. You made this work possible.

I never thought corrections would be the highlight reel of my career. But it was. The stories will go on without me—but for now, this is where I set down my pen.

Thanks, Oakwood Correctional Facility.

www.ingramcontent.com/pod-product-compliance
Lightning Source LLC
LaVergne TN
LVHW050815061126
851857LV00012B/809
* 9 7 9 8 9 9 7 0 6 7 7 0 0 *